A PLAGUE UPON OUR HOUSE

MY FIGHT AT THE
TRUMP WHITE HOUSE TO STOP COVID
FROM DESTROYING AMERICA

A PLAGUE UPON OUR HOUSE

MY FIGHT AT THE TRUMP WHITE HOUSE TO STOP COVID FROM DESTROYING AMERICA

Liberatio
Protocol

SCOTT W. ATLAS, MD

A LIBERATIO PROTOCOL BOOK

An Imprint of Post Hill Press

ISBN: 978-1-63758-220-6

ISBN (eBook): 978-1-63758-221-3

A Plague Upon Our House:

My Fight at the Trump White House to Stop COVID from Destroying America

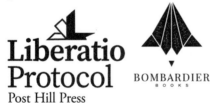

Liberatio Protocol
Post Hill Press

New York • Nashville

posthillpress.com

Published in the United States of America

1 2 3 4 5 6 7 8 9 10

DEDICATION

To Ali,
the toughest person I have ever known.
You were there when I needed you most. You still are, and I still do.

***

In special remembrance of all those who lost loved ones,
and to all those still suffering from the failures of those in power.
May you find some peace in knowing that the truth will prevail.
And may we all never let this happen again.

***

In loving memory of my dad.
You would have said the truth, directly to their faces, just like I did.
I hope you watched.

TABLE OF CONTENTS

ACKNOWLEDGMENTS

- To our children and young people, who are the reason I became involved. I know many of you are still confused and suffering from misguided, incompetent, and unethical leadership. Stay strong!

- To the thousands of wonderful people who contacted me, many of you more than once, from all over the country and the world—the mothers, fathers, grandparents, nine-to-five and midnight shift workers, students, professors, clergy, teachers, business owners, taxi drivers, NIH scientists, restaurant workers, doctors, and more—far too many to list. Because of your heartfelt support and encouragement, I was never going to give up speaking the truth, no matter what.

- To Jay, Martin, and Sunetra. We are bonded for life. I am honored to call you friends and colleagues. We were right about everything, and they know it. We will never, never, never stop speaking the truth. That, too, we know.

- To John Ioannidis. I am so grateful for your counsel and friendship. I cannot thank you enough for your unending encouragement and wisdom. Critical thinking matters, yes it does.

- To my incredible White House buddies for everything, especially for being there when I needed you (every day)—John Rader, Derek Lyons, and Liz Horning. That was insane!! We fought the fight, together.

- To my phenomenal data partners who worked under pressure 24/7 to provide me real-time stats on demand and far more than that: Jennifer Cabrera, Len Cabrera, Mills Carter, Clayton, Karl Dierenbach, Aaron Ginn, Jessica Gordon, Justin Hart, Nathan Hyatt, A. J. Kay, Phil Kerpen, Kyle Lamb, Todd Lowdon, Megan Mansell, Ian Miller, Alex Rodriguez, Joshua Stevenson, Jon R. Taylor, Sara T., Andy Bostom, and many others too numerous to list. Thank you so much. The nation heard your words, saw your charts, and benefitted from your labors.

- Speaking of charts in this book: Ian Miller! Fantastic! Thank you again.

- To my colleagues at Hoover, especially Victor Davis Hanson and John Cochrane, who rose up for me for the right reasons. Leadership is shown by action. Proud to have you as my colleagues.

- To the thousands of doctors and scientists from all over the world who also stood up for scientific truth and against incompetence and tyranny. It's a battle, and you are an inspiration. Never give up, this is not over.

- To Abir Ballan and Nick Hudson. Thank you for your unending commitment in the face of adversity and censorship. I am grateful for your friendship.

- To the hundreds of people who took the time to approach me personally in Washington with support. Your kindness and encouragement were more important than you realize. I won't forget it.

- To the many scientists and researchers who sent me their excellent work during this pandemic. I am so sorry that I didn't have the bandwidth to reply in more detail, or to coauthor or edit pieces with you, or even, at times, to reply at all to your kind emails. But I read every single one and learned from you.

- To Kayleigh McEnany, Douglas Sellers, Madison Porter, and Johnny McEntee. You proved there were rational people there—I needed that!

- To several very special governors, senators, and congressmen. I learned much from all our discussions and even more from your leadership in the face of adversity. Our country needs your courage and honesty. Without that, the whole thing is finished.

- To my neuroradiology colleagues and former trainees from all over the world who contacted me to express trust and support—thank you; it mattered!

- To the journalists with integrity whom I came to know. It was a great pleasure to talk thoughtfully with you about the pandemic. Your challenging questions helped me think through what was important.

- To the White House Secret Service and security staff who always kept it safe and secure with the utmost professionalism, from the East Wing to the West Wing and on the Lawns. Thank you for everything you do.

- To the fair journalist at the most dishonest network on cable TV. Your supportive email when I was publicly named as advisor to the president—"I'm pleased to see you in the mix on the nation's response to the virus. *Data*!!!"—was appreciated. As promised, I won't reveal your name, because you need your paycheck.

- To Mickael. You made it feel like a home. Thank you for taking care of me and for your warnings about DC.

- To Grace. You may not realize it, but your support when I came home was really important.

- To John Yoo, my friend and much more, and Dee Pugh. Thank you both for your wisdom.

- To my great editor, Adam Bellow, and agent, Jonathan Bronitsky. Thank you for tolerating my rants and emotions while reliving the total insanity of it all.

"Truth is incontrovertible. Panic may resent it. Ignorance may deride it. Malice may distort it. But there it is."

—*Winston Churchill*

INTRODUCTION
A Broken Trust

No book about the SARS2 coronavirus pandemic can be written without first stating that it has been a great tragedy. Around the world, at the time of this writing, four million deaths have been tallied. More than 600,000 American deaths have been attributed directly to the virus. We realize the blessing that this virus generally spared the young and healthy. We also recognize that the death toll is inaccurate. None of that matters to those who lost loved ones. Countless lives will also have been lost due to the missteps of those we entrusted with working for the public good. Directly from the lockdowns, missed medical care; school closures; massive economic strains; incalculable psychological damage, especially to young people; and a worldwide humanitarian crisis will burden us for decades. While inflicting enormous harm, the lockdowns also failed to protect the vulnerable.

*   *   *   *   *

As I finish this book, I am hopeful that we are seeing the light at the end of a long tunnel. Deaths are not likely to rise dramatically when cases sharply increase, a different pattern than in the initial waves. That "decoupling" between cases and deaths would be to a great extent due to the successful vaccination of those at risk to die. Unfortunately, it is unlikely the recurring hysteria and mismanagement by those in power will end so quickly. After more than eighteen months of experience, there remains an almost bizarre lack of understanding that the virus will not simply disappear. Instead, on its way to becoming endemic, cases will continue to peak and ebb periodically, as they have done and continue to do in characteristic cycles all over the world and regionally in the United States. We must learn to live with the virus by offering vaccines to the vulnerable, aggressively exploring early treatments, while also accepting some risk, rather than employing failed, harmful restrictions on low-risk people every time the pattern recurs. Instead of recognizing the evidence, the flow of misleading information lacking perspective, policies counter to scientific data, and the absence of transparency continue:

- The unscientific obsession with stopping all cases of COVID-19 continues, including the variants that all scientists expected as the virus mutates and becomes less lethal, without acknowledging the low risk for the overwhelming majority and what should be today's protection of the most vulnerable to death.

- Accountability remains absent from government leaders, public health officials, and scientists in failing to admit errors about lockdowns; some even distort their records and portray disastrous death tallies as "successes."

- The CDC and public health leaders still fail to visibly acknowledge and then educate the public about the natural immunity in recovered COVID patients or to incorporate that biological fact into our nation's vaccine policies. The public needs to know that data continues to accrue showing natural immunity after SARS2 infection, like other infectious diseases, is probably superior to vaccine-related protection.

- Public health officials and government leaders keep using wildly incorrect projections that instill fear and alarm the public, and when they're wrong, they fail to acknowledge this fact.

- Our public health recommendations on masks and distancing did not change after scientific data showed previous rules were arbitrary, incorrect, and ineffective. As this was written, the CDC abruptly reissued another call for masking, even after vaccination, despite the lack of scientific data to support it. Many schools force children to wear masks, contrary to very clear science and simple logic. Must we prove the earth is round again?

- Serious problems with the data, including overcounting of COVID as the cause of many hospitalizations and deaths in the United States, have never been explained to the public and acknowledged, even though it has been documented in the medical literature.

- There continue to be delays in clinical trials and approvals of safe, widely available drugs that show potential efficacy in clinical reports, as if vaccination is the only option.

- A COVID testing requirement has been imposed in schools and university campuses, grossly violating ethical standards, including the CDC's own statement only months ago in late 2020 that "it is both unethical and illegal to test someone who doesn't want to be tested, including students whose parents or guardians do not want them to be tested."

- The spirit if not the letter of informed consent has been violated with a vaccine clinical trial in young children who have extremely low risk from the illness and rarely spread it.

- The nation still awaits any indication that there will be a full investigation into the origin of the deadly virus, even if it uncovers potential corruption in our nation's top science agencies and public health leaders. The world is owed full exposure without delay.

Why do these failures persist in a nominally science-based, freethinking, and ethical society like ours? Is the herd mentality so powerful, is fear such a dominant emotion, that all critical thinking and values disappear? If the US tallies 50,000 deaths from COVID next year, will we accept that with the relaxed attitude we have about the flu, which has that death toll every year? If not, why not? Are we a nation of science or science-deniers? Do we demand accountability and learn from past error? Is this country committed to the free exchange of ideas, so that truth is determined by evidence and debate rather than decree and false declarations of consensus? Do facts still matter? And what is the end-point, an endless series of panic-driven lockdowns or finally a recognition that the virus will become endemic? Are we committed to civil liberties? The answers to these questions are profoundly consequential.

One issue stands above all others—the urgent need to restore trust in our vital institutions. The management of this pandemic has left a stain on many of America's once noble institutions, including our elite universities, research institutes and journals, and public health agencies. Earning it back will not be easy:

Trust in government. Almost all governors made entirely arbitrary distinctions. Even if one believed in the health benefits of these diktats, they were handed down with shocking disregard for the potential damages and deaths. In addition to seeing convincing data to justify such measures in the future, the citizenry must be convinced that rules apply to everyone. When elected officials are caught enjoying indoor dining with lobbyists, or public health leaders ignore their own restrictions on family gatherings, they undermine the moral legitimacy necessary for voluntary compliance. That puts the rule of law in future emergencies at risk.

Trust in public health leadership. There has been a repeated, erratic discussion coming from public health officials. On masks, America's leading voice of public health issued a number of statements over a period of months that were in direct conflict with each other and with the data, and he still fails to recognize the most compelling studies. On testing, the CDC put up a guideline, then changed it, then took it down, then put back something close to the original. There was no science to prompt those changes. The most visible face of public health praised four northeast US states with the highest rate of fatalities for following his guidance, despite their deadly performance. We also saw statements and actions from our top health and medical agencies that undermined trust in vaccines and potential treatments, an extremely important part of saving lives in the next pandemic.

Trust in science. The pandemic exposed grave problems with the essential functioning of science, research and debate. Elite research universities, public health agencies, and top scientific journals quickly fell in line with herd thinking about the pandemic. Instead of open and free discourse to seek the scientific truths underlying urgently needed solutions, we have seen silencing, censoring, and slandering of scientists whose interpretations differed from the desired narrative. Prestigious journals are now openly contaminated with politics. Academia and the research community, dominated by a single viewpoint, actively engage in intimidation and false declarations of consensus, as well as through abuse of the peer-review system. That intolerance has fostered a climate of fear and inhibited other scientists and health experts from contributing to the discussion, effectively inducing self-censorship. This dangerous trend threatens the free exchange of ideas essential to democracy.

Trust in educational leaders. The priorities of teachers and their unions were exposed as self-centered, driven by fear for the adult teachers, most of whom are at very low risk, at the expense of the health and future of children. The same holds true for our university leadership. Children are not to be used as shields for adults. No longer can we, as parents and concerned citizens, permit coerced injections of experimental drugs and required testing for access to university education. These requirements are not only unscientific, they also violate our nation's long-established standards for ethical conduct, medical privacy, and autonomy over one's own body.

Trust in fellow citizens. Policymakers in concert with the elite class inflicted great harm by undermining fundamental trust in our fellow citizens. Elites in the media have made "freedom" a selfish idea and politicized dissent on the efficacy of masks or various potential treatments. Restrictions on liberty were also destructive by inflaming class distinctions with their differential impact: exposing essential workers, sacrificing low-income families and kids, destroying single-parent homes, and eviscerating small businesses, while at the same time large companies were bailed out, elites worked from home with barely an interruption, and the ultra-rich got richer, leveraging their bully pulpit to demonize and cancel those who challenged their preferred policy options.

This book is written with several purposes in mind. First, it will serve as an important part of the historical record of the greatest health care crisis in the past century—the pandemic and its management. The four-month period during my service as advisor to the president of the United States will provide a candid perspective on how our leaders functioned in this crisis, without the distorting lenses of the media and politics. Second, it will clarify the facts underlying the pandemic, free from the filter of government bureaucrats, academics, and scientists with political and other biases. Third, it will expose profound issues in our society that could interfere with our ability to address future crises and threaten the very principles of freedom and order that we often take for granted and that the rest of the world depends on.

The reader should feel confident of two certainties. One is that every word in this book, every event described, every statement quoted, is absolutely true. The second is that several people described in this book will vehemently deny its truth. That is expected, not only because they will have been exposed in the light of day, beyond the protection of their media allies, but also because we have already witnessed their behavior with regard to truth. We should know who to trust by now.

In considering all the surprising events that unfolded in this past year, two in particular stand out. I have been shocked at the enormous power of government officials to unilaterally decree a sudden and severe shutdown of society—to simply close businesses and schools by edict, restrict personal movements, mandate behavior, regulate inter-actions with our family members, and eliminate our most basic free-doms, without any defined end and with little accountability.

And I remain stunned at the acceptance by the American peo-ple of draconian rules, restrictions, and unprecedented mandates, even those that are arbitrary, destructive, and wholly unscientific. The acquiescence of the citizenry to such extraordinary and ill-con-ceived restrictions in a nation that was founded on the principles of freedom from an overbearing government, in a country that stands as the world's beacon for independence and liberty, is nothing less than shocking.

Today, after all that we have endured from this pandemic, we still must ask why so few were willing to speak out when the most disastrous health policies in history were foisted on ordinary people and above all on our children, our country's most precious resource. We all should ask:

- Where were the scientists?

- Where were the economists?

- Where were the pediatricians and psychologists?

- Where were the teachers and university leaders?

- Where were the investigative journalists?

- Where were the constitutional lawyers?

- Where were the human rights advocates?

- Where were the ethicists?

- Where were the independent Americans?

At this point, one could make a reasonable case that those who consider reintroducing significant societal restrictions without ac-knowledging their failures and serious harms are putting forth dan-gerous misinformation. But I will not call for their official rebuke or punishment. I will not try to cancel them. I will not try to extin-guish their opinions. And I will not lie to distort their words and defame them. To do so would repeat a behavior of intimidating the discourse that is critical to educating the public and arriving at the scientific truths we desperately need.

This crisis has also exposed what we all know has existed for years but have tolerated in this country—the overt bias of the media, the lack of diverse viewpoints on campuses, the absence of neutrality in controlling social media, and now more visibly than ever the intrusion of politics into science. Ultimately, the freedom to seek the truth and openly state it is at risk.

The United States is on the precipice of losing its cherished freedoms, with censorship and cancellation of all those who bring views forward that differ from the "accepted mainstream." It is not clear if our democracy, with its defining freedoms, will fully recover, even after we survive the pandemic itself. But it is clear that people must step up—meaning speak up, as we are allowed, as we are expected to do in free societies—or it has no chance.

In 1841, Charles Mackay presciently spoke about the herd mentality: "Men, it has been well said, think in herds; it will be seen that they go mad in herds, while they only recover their senses slowly, and one by one."

So how do we proceed at this very moment, in this country, with its heavily damaged psyche? Those of us who want the truth must keep seeking it, and those of us who see the truth must keep speaking it. *Because truth matters.*

CHAPTER 1
America off the Rails

It was February 2020, and for weeks I had been trying to finish my book on reforming the US health care system. I was under pressure to meet an impending deadline necessitated by the upcoming election, which I thought would center on single-payer health care. My focus was compiling data on the issues most poorly understood: single-payer health care, the public option, reforming Medicare, and improving health care quality and access for the poor. The failures of the Affordable Care Act seemed to generate a significant momentum toward all-out single payer rather than a reexamination of the causes of those failures and the consequences of the increased government regulations imposed by the ACA.

As always, I needed to be thorough and accurate. But this time more was at stake. Like many issues, health care reform had often been argued on emotion and with disregard for the evidence. I kept focusing on the final slide that I had used for years at Stanford's Hoover Institution to end every one of my lectures: Facts Matter.

Like most people who spent most of their days on a computer, my tendency was to flip back and forth to other things on the internet, as a quick break from my own work. News accounts had been describing increasingly alarming information about a deadly new virus emanating from Wuhan, China. Separate from my general concern about the spread of the infection, I was confused about some of the basic numbers being aired. The overall message about the virus coming out of the World Health Organization (WHO) seemed to have obvious flaws. To my mind, the extremely high risk estimates seemed very misleading. The reported fatality rates were based only on patients who were sick enough to seek medical care rather than on the undoubtedly much larger population of infected individuals. I was stunned that this basic methodological flaw was being overlooked by almost everyone, while the exaggerated fatality rate of 3.4 percent was highlighted throughout the media. Every legitimate medical scientist should have called that out. I was puzzled at their silence.

In the United States and throughout the world, a naive discussion about statistical models ensued. To an extraordinary and unprecedented extent, these epidemiological models were featured front and center in news headlines, with no perspective on their usefulness. I simply presumed that every serious academic researcher understood the role and limitations of such models, particularly how the wide range of assumptions that go into them can dramatically impact their predictions. Reminiscent of other legendary frenzies in history, like the tulip bulb mania or the tech stock bubble, hypothetical extreme-risk scenarios went seemingly unchallenged and were given absolute credence in the media.

At the same time, common sense and well established principles of medicine were being ignored. Every second-year medical student knew that the elderly were almost certainly the most vulnerable group of people, since they were virtually always at highest risk of death and serious consequences from respiratory infections. Yet this was not stressed. To the contrary, the implication of reports and the public faces of official expertise implied that everyone was equally in danger. Even the initial evidence showed that elderly, frail people with preexisting comorbidities—conditions that weakened their natural immunological defenses—were the ones at highest risk of death. This was a historical fact shared by other respiratory viruses, including seasonal influenza. The one unusual feature of this virus was the fact that children had an extraordinarily low risk. Yet this positive and reassuring news was never emphasized. Instead, with total disregard of the evidence of selective risk consistent with other respiratory viruses, public health officials recommended draconian isolation of everyone.

The architects of the American lockdown strategy were Dr. Anthony Fauci and Dr. Deborah Birx. With Dr. Robert Redfield, the director of the CDC, they were the most influential medical members of the White House Coronavirus Task Force.

The Task Force at its January inception consisted of a small group assembled by President Trump that was coordinated through the National Security Council and advised by several US government agencies and science advisors. At its onset, the group was chaired by Health and Human Services Secretary Alex Azar. Other members included Robert O'Brien, assistant to the president for National Security Affairs; Dr. Robert Redfield, director of the Centers for Disease Control and Prevention; Dr. Anthony Fauci, director of the National Institute of Allergy and Infectious Diseases at the National Institutes of Health; Deputy Secretary Stephen Biegun, Department of State; Ken Cuccinelli, acting deputy secretary, Department of Homeland Security; Joel Szabat, acting under secretary for policy, Department of Transportation; Matthew Pottinger, assistant to the president and deputy national security advisor; Rob Blair, assistant to the president and senior advisor to the chief of staff; Joseph Grogan, assistant to the president and director of the Domestic Policy Council; Christopher Liddell, assistant to the president and deputy chief of staff for policy coordination; and Derek Kan, executive associate director, Office of Management and Budget. It was formally announced by the press secretary on January 29, 2020, with a statement that directly reflected the views of Dr. Anthony Fauci. It read in part: "The risk of infection for Americans remains low, and all agencies are working aggressively to monitor this continuously evolving situation and to keep the public informed."

The Task Force quickly expanded over the next month to include a new chairman, Vice President Pence. The White House also announced that Dr. Deborah Birx would be the Task Force coordinator. Birx had worked in the State Department as the US AIDS coordinator under the Obama and Trump administrations—

hence she was often addressed by the honorific "ambassador." She had been working in the government since 1985. In the February 26 announcement by the White House, others were added to the Task Force, including Secretary of the Treasury Steven Mnuchin, Surgeon General Jerome Adams, and National Economic Council Director Larry Kudlow. The Task Force ultimately included representation from numerous federal agencies concerned with health, science, national emergencies and logistics, the economy, and many other relevant concerns.

The Task Force dealt with a number of issues at its origin. Since the country had not been well prepared for a pandemic, one of the primary tasks was to develop adequate testing, the mainstay of public health in early infectious disease outbreaks. The second main set of tasks centered around production and logistics of supportive medical equipment, including ventilators, personal protective supplies for hospitals, and extra beds and personnel to accommodate sick patients anticipated to overwhelm the system.

Dr. Birx, Dr. Redfield, and Dr. Fauci—often called "the nation's expert in infectious disease"—dominated all discussions about the health and medical aspects of the emerging pandemic. One thing was very clear—all three were cut from the same cloth. First, they were all bureaucrats, sharing a background that crossed paths in government agencies. Second, they shared a long history in HIV/AIDS as a public health crisis. Almost the entire background of both Dr. Birx and Dr. Redfield was in HIV/AIDS. That was problematic, because HIV couldn't be more different from SARS2 in its biology, its amenability to testing and contact tracing, its spread, and the implications of those facts for its control. Indeed, the three of them spent many years focusing on the development of a vaccine, rather than treatment, for HIV/AIDS—a vaccine that still does not exist.

It's also worth noting the very relevant history of Dr. Fauci in regard to AIDS. He created headlines in *New York Times*, UPI, and AP articles for his alarmist speculations in his 1983 *JAMA* editorial that AIDS could be transmitted by "routine close contact, as within a family household." It had already been known that transmission was via fluids through blood or sexual contact. Less than two months later, on June 26 in the *Baltimore Sun*, Fauci publicly contradicted his own explosive claim. "It is absolutely preposterous to suggest that AIDS can be contracted through normal social contact like being in the same room with someone or sitting on a bus with them. The poor gays have received a very raw deal on this." That seemed like quite a flip-flop, with no new evidence or explanation given—more reminiscent of a politician than a reliable scientist.

Most others on the Task Force were juggling several concerns and had no medical background. This was one more responsibility added to their portfolios, so they deferred to those deemed medical experts. Drs. Birx and Fauci commandeered federal policy under President Trump and publicly advocated for a total societal shutdown. Instead of focusing on protecting the most vulnerable, their illogical and extraordinarily blunt response with predictable, wide-ranging harms had been instituted as though it were simple common sense.

Over those first several weeks, fear had taken hold of the public. Media commentators and even many policy experts, many of whom had no perspective on health care, were filling the airwaves and opinion pages with naive and incorrect predictions. This misinformation was going unchecked, and was indeed repeatedly endorsed and sensationalized in the media. Some whom I had previously considered among my smartest colleagues and friends expressed great confusion and a striking absence of logic in analyzing what was happening.

I asked myself, "Where are the critical thinkers?"

As a health policy researcher for more than fifteen years with decades in medical science and data analysis, I had never seen such flawed thinking. I was bewildered at the lack of logic, the absence of common sense, and the reliance on fundamentally flawed science. Suddenly, computer modelers and people without any perspective about clinical illnesses were dominating the airwaves. Along with millions of Americans, I began witnessing unprecedented responses from those in power and nonscientific recommendations by public health spokespeople: societal lockdowns including business and school closures, stay-at-home restrictions on individual movements, and arbitrary decrees by local, state, and federal governments. These recommendations were not just based on panic; they were responsible for generating even more panic. COVID had rapidly become the most important health policy crisis in a century. My policy book on the merits of a competition-based health system simply had to wait.

*   *   *   *   *

Over February and early March, I dedicated myself to studying the pandemic in detail to understand and generate the appropriate policy prescriptions. The more I studied the data and the literature, the more obvious it became that basic biology and simple logic were missing from the discussion. Instead, fear had seemingly displaced critical thinking about the data already at hand. No one seemed to remember many fundamentals of science taught in college and medical school. I began asking myself, "Where are the rational scientists?"

I soon found one. Dr. John Ioannidis, one of the world's most renowned epidemiologists and a colleague previously unknown to me at Stanford University, authored an amazingly prescient piece in March entitled, "A Fiasco in the Making? As the Coronavirus Pandemic Takes Hold, We Are Making Decisions without Reliable Data." His short essay will go down as one of the most important— and most infamously ignored—publications in modern medical science.

Ioannidis began with what should have been obvious to all critical thinkers with any medical knowledge. His key points:

- "Reported case fatality rates, like the official 3.4% rate from the World Health Organization, cause horror—and are meaningless. Patients who have been tested for SARS-CoV-2 are disproportionately those with severe symptoms and bad outcomes."

- "The data collected so far on how many people are infected and how the epidemic is evolving are utterly unreliable…and probably the vast majority of infections due to SARS-CoV-2 are being missed."

He went on to list some very preliminary estimates with simple statistics, implied by a *Diamond Princess* cruise ship that had been carrying an early group infected with the virus, a closed population, all of whom were tested:

- "The case fatality rate there was 1.0%, but this was a largely elderly population, in which the death rate from Covid-19 is much higher. Projecting the *Diamond Princess* mortality rate onto the age structure of the U.S. population, the death rate among people infected with Covid-19 would be 0.125%. But since this estimate is based on extremely thin data…the real death rate could stretch from five times lower (0.025%) to five times higher (0.625%)…. Adding these extra sources of uncertainty, reasonable estimates for the case fatality ratio in the general U.S. population vary from 0.05% to 1%."

Prophetically, Ioannidis also pointed out what would be one of the most egregious failures of the world's public health agencies and "experts," including the CDC, the leaders of the White House Task Force, and countless others. He refuted an inexplicably simplistic reliance on a positive virus test as causation of death—naive thinking that has persisted to the time of this writing and has likely caused massive errors in death counts in this pandemic. He again stated the obvious:

- "A positive test for coronavirus does not mean necessarily that this virus is always primarily responsible for a patient's demise," and "in some people who die from viral respiratory pathogens, more than one virus is found upon autopsy and bacteria are often superimposed."

Ioannidis also noted that other viruses in the same coronavirus family already circulate, a key fact that should have indicated at least the possibility of some preexisting immune protection in the population.

In his call for more data-based thinking, Ioannidis documented that we did not have evidence that social distancing, school closures, stay-at-home orders, and lockdowns worked, and noted they might even be harmful: "In the absence of data, prepare-for-the-worst reasoning leads to extreme measures of social distancing and lockdowns. Unfortunately, we do not know if these measures work." Citing evidence to the contrary in an extensive review by Oxford University's Center for Evidence-Based Medicine, he observed: "School closures, for example, may reduce transmission rates. But they may also backfire if children socialize anyhow, if school closure leads children to spend more time with susceptible elderly family members, if children at home disrupt their parents' ability to work, and more."

Ioannidis also pointed out the simple biological fact that isolating young, healthy people with no significant risk for serious illness would reduce the chances of developing herd immunity, a biological phenomenon that protects the population and prevents death in high-risk individuals.

Standing virtually alone in the United States back in mid-March of 2020, Ioannidis warned with astounding accuracy about the catastrophic health harms and devastating impacts of an extended lockdown:

> …the extra deaths may not be due to coronavirus but to other common diseases and conditions such as heart attacks, strokes, trauma, bleeding, and the like that are not adequately treated" and "we don't know how long social distancing measures and lockdowns can be maintained without major consequences to the economy, society, and mental health. Unpredictable evolutions may ensue, including financial crisis, unrest, civil strife, war, and

a meltdown of the social fabric. At a minimum, we need unbiased prevalence and incidence data for the evolving infectious load to guide decision-making…with lockdowns of months, if not years, life largely stops, short-term and long-term consequences are entirely unknown, and billions, not just millions, of lives may be eventually at stake."

I vividly remember my relief at discovering that someone else had understood what I was ranting about to my family every night at dinner. Yet despite his prescient observations, now proven correct, the Ioannidis article was met with massive pushback and irresponsible claims from other academic epidemiologists. Professors at esteemed institutions painted the internationally respected scholar as dangerous. For example, Dr. Marc Lipsitch, an epidemiology professor at the Harvard T.H. Chan School of Public Health, was reported by the *Washington Post* to have expressed "bafflement" at Ioannidis's essay. As a harbinger of what would follow from the scientific community who delegitimized and villainized experts with differing views, Lipsitch used straw-man arguments. "We had enough evidence to see that uncontrolled spread was very dangerous…the idea that we should just sort of sit by and gather data calmly struck me as incredibly naïve," warned Lipsitch, a shameful distortion of what Ioannidis actually wrote.

I knew otherwise. What Ioannidis had written was far from baffling. It was sensible, straightforward, logical, and factual. Any medical student who had stayed awake during lectures about virus infections and immunology should have understood and agreed with Ioannidis. And nowhere did he advocate that we "sit by" and observe "uncontrolled spread." He simply recognized some of the potential harms of lockdown measures and cited data to question their effectiveness. Noting the potential harm of lockdowns is not the same as advocating a "let it rip" strategy, as any fair-minded person knows. At that time, though, I myself was still naive about the search for truth in universities.

*   *   *   *   *

That spring, I began writing and speaking publicly to clarify the facts about the data and the appropriate direction of policies. I was stunned that some very smart people were citing the overtly flawed, misleading statistics that had been repeated virtually everywhere in the media. There were so many gross errors and misinterpretations of the data that it was going to be difficult to overcome the false narratives that had already taken hold.

It was not just that this was my field of expertise as a health policy scholar; it was my obligation as a doctor and a citizen to state the facts and put forth solutions to minimize the harms already spiraling out of control. While the virus was spreading widely, its fatality rate had been wildly exaggerated, simply by looking at the cruise ship with the first outbreak, the *Diamond Princess*. The media was highlighting severely flawed British and other epidemiological models that used worst-case scenarios and disregarded basic principles of acquired immunity seen in every other pandemic, falsely claiming many millions of Americans would die without a lockdown. Even though there was still tremendous uncertainty, common sense about isolating the sick, prioritizing testing, and protecting those known to be high-risk had been abandoned in favor of panic and shutting down everything.

Despite what Ioannidis had written, several fear-provoking claims about the coronavirus were becoming ingrained in the public mind. These false claims had been initiated by the WHO but were amplified by a constant drumbeat from epidemiologists and others in the public limelight:

- This SARS2 coronavirus is extraordinarily deadly, far more deadly than the flu by several orders of magnitude.

- Virtually everyone is at high risk to die.

- No one has any immunity, because this virus is entirely new,

- Everyone is dangerous and spreads the infection.

- Asymptomatic people are major drivers of the spread.

- Testing virtually everyone is urgently needed, and all those testing positive should be isolated.

- Locking down everyone is essential—closing schools and businesses, confining people to their homes, and isolating everyone from others and even their own family members is urgently needed.

- Everyone should wear masks, because masks will protect everyone and stop the spread.

- The only protection is from a vaccine, and that is years away.

By late March, methodically detailing the evidence in a rational way became urgent. Fundamental science and straightforward logic were being routinely denied by public health officials and news show guests labeled as experts. The advice of Dr. Fauci, Dr. Birx, and others had led to an unprecedented imposition of extreme measures by state governors from coast to coast. That included school closures and severe lockdowns whose harms would be almost unthinkable, especially on lower-income families and the poor.

In response to those misleading claims about the virus propagated by the WHO, the CDC, and others, the public was easily convinced about the urgency of shutting down—at least temporarily. The draconian measures were acceptable, primarily because they were sold as short-term measures. A fifteen-day hold to make sure hospitals were ready to treat the anticipated inflow of COVID patients without being overwhelmed seemed very sensible—especially to the American public who had seen reports of ventilator shortages and bedlam in Italian hospitals.

Fears were also stoked by the unpreparedness of the nation with regard to testing. The CDC had first developed a test in January, but as a harbinger of follies to come, glitches delayed its use. That also delayed availability of tests produced by private sector laboratories, and that was followed by delays in testing turnaround and other issues. The HHS inspector general issued a report in April 2020, criticizing that debacle. The lack of tests "limited hospitals' ability to monitor the health of patients and staff," the inspector general concluded. As complicated as massive real-time testing needs under a new pandemic might be, the erratic start and the ensuing blame game between Secretary Azar, testing czar Brett Giroir, and the states worsened the panic and added veracity to the claims of incompetence.

Feeling frightened, even a little panicked at the lack of simple common sense, I realized this was now an enormous problem. That said, I never even considered that it would be controversial to lay out the contrary evidence. In my own career, consideration of evidence was not only usual, it was essential to arrive at a correct diagnosis and treatment of the problem. That was literally always the way it worked in medicine and science. This time, the need for fact was more obvious and urgent than ever.

Perhaps the most fundamental error that went unchallenged was the World Health Organization's initial characterization of this virus as entirely new. Even its name—novel coronavirus—implied that we knew nothing about it in terms of its causes, effects, and management protocols. That "novelty" also implied that no one would have any immune-system protection from it.

On its face, that depiction was misleading. As Dr. Ioannidis and every virology textbook stated, the world already had decades of experience with coronaviruses—including at least four "endemic" ones in circulation today. That mischaracterization helped incite panic and was fundamental to prompting the ensuing draconian lockdowns.

* * * * *

In late March 2020, I began speaking out against lockdowns. Since I usually submitted my op-eds myself without the help of the Hoover Institution media staff, I shot one to the *Wall Street Journal*. It was quickly rejected, with a polite "several pieces in the works addressing various aspects of this"—though none did. Because I felt a bit of panic about the dark road we were headed down, I wanted to get this out ASAP. The *New York Times* had already published a similar piece by Dr. David Katz, a former director of Yale's Disease Prevention Center, so that was out. The Hoover staff suggested the *Washington Times* for a quick publication, and they were right

In that publication, I echoed the sensible strategy of Ioannidis and put forth the idea of "targeted protection" as an alternative to the widespread societal closures. By then, those shutdowns had already been implemented in many states across the country, based on the advice of Drs. Fauci and Birx, the architects and main advocates of the American lockdown strategy. Scandalous failures of protecting the nursing home population, who were known to be the most at-risk and who were already living in a highly regulated, confined environment, should have already prompted a change in strategy. That strategy, even back in spring 2020, was not only failing to prevent the elderly from dying, it was also already leading to enormous, readily apparent health harms by preventing serious medical care to adults and children.

I wrote, "There is a different strategy, one focused on protecting the vulnerable, self-isolating the mildly sick, and limiting group interactions." Drawing from the Ioannidis essay and *the New York Times* piece by Katz, I stressed two important points: "1) targeted isolation is correct policy in terms of medical science, not just economically; and 2) testing is important but it should be prioritized, instead of thought of as urgent for everyone." I tried to point out that it was not "lives versus economics" when one chose between lockdowns and targeted protection – it was all about lives. And as part of the targeted strategy, I listed testing prioritizations straight out of the Infectious Diseases Society of America recommendations at the time.

During the preparation of that piece, I contacted John Ioannidis. Although we both worked at Stanford, we didn't know each other. We discussed the data and the research in detail. We were on the exact same page. During our first phone conversation, I expressed shock and dismay at the lack of simple logic about the virus. Always the optimist, Ioannidis uttered what would become his trademark encouragement. "Don't worry, Scott. The truth will prevail!"

At around the same time, I delivered an early policy briefing to my colleagues and others at Hoover. Again, I stressed protecting the elderly, instead of widespread lockdowns, and I recommended using safety measures like masks "for when you are close to people, like crowded places." I explained that the WHO's projected fatality rate of 3.4 percent was highly misleading and likely to be an overestimate.

In April, I published several opinion pieces in *The Hill* that pointed out the severe potential health harms from the hospital shutdowns. Over two dozen states and many hospitals had stopped "non-essential" procedures and surgery. This was a misleading way to cast it—it was often very important, very serious medical care. That move also introduced even more fear into patients who stopped seeking non-COVID care, and it compounded the damage from the total isolation policies that had been implemented. In these pieces, I stressed targeted protection, including increased prioritization of the elderly by testing to help protect them. Considering the tremendous harms of locking down society, I went so far as to propose testing for immunity—although it was not clear how costly that testing might be—as a way to open society safely, as a "temporary" maneuver. Even by then, millions of Americans had natural immunity from having survived the infection.

Over the end of March and first half of April, I also conducted about ten media interviews, responding to requests from radio, TV, and podcasts interested in a commonsense articulation of the situation that differed from the general narrative. My main points were that targeted protection made sense, not broad lockdowns, especially given that the elderly harbored a far higher risk than younger, healthier people; that children had an extremely low risk; and that the lockdowns and school closures were already enormously harmful.

The next publication that impacted me dramatically was research that also came out of Stanford. This study, first published on

April 14, 2020, tested people in Santa Clara County for antibodies to the virus. By their "seroprevalence" data of SARS-CoV-2 antibodies, epidemiologists Dr. Eran Bendavid and his coauthors, including Ioannidis and Jay Bhattacharya, calculated that the infection may be far more widespread—about fifty times more widespread—than indicated by the number of "confirmed" cases. That meant that the reported fatality rates were grossly off-base, too high by a factor of fifty. It was soon followed by another piece reaching the same conclusion.

The Stanford study was met with harsh blowback from both a large segment of the scientific community and the lay press. Yet another attempt to delegitimize researchers who countered the mainstream narrative ensued. False accusations of bias based on research funding by these exceptional scientists caused a frenzy. In the first of many shameful actions during this pandemic, Stanford University faculty members attempted to discredit, and effectively censor, the findings. They even participated in an unprecedented call for internal investigation. The details behind who initiated that investigation remain hidden at the time of this writing, other than its bottom line conclusion—complete vindication of the study and its authors.

Around this time, I exchanged the first of what became almost daily emails and calls with Dr. Jay Bhattacharya. Our backgrounds are overlapping, as both of us are health policy scholars as well as medical scientists at Stanford. Even though we superficially knew each other, we had never worked together. On campus, we had met in the past during health policy seminars. Jay had seen my Hoover briefing on the pandemic, as well as some other things I had written and discussed in interviews.

Jay began by expressing his strong support, saying, "Scott, everything you are saying is correct, keep saying it!" We discussed with horror the irrational nature of the response to the pandemic. We commiserated about how well-established, fundamental knowledge about infections and immunity had been ignored. We also talked about how the environment was hostile, shockingly so, from people in science and medicine. I didn't yet fully grasp the level of venom from scientists already wedded, in such an unscientific and emotional manner, to the narrative of lockdowns. At that point, I had conducted only about a dozen interviews based on my published writings. But I was stunned, especially by the apparent attempt to censor research at Stanford. We vowed to stay in contact, not realizing that would later turn into near daily conversations and ultimately into the closest of friendships. With characteristic optimism, he said, "Don't worry, Scott, we are right; the truth will come out. History will show it."

My next piece turned everything on its head for me. "The Data Is In—Stop the Panic and End the Total Isolation" was published that same month in *The Hill*. I pointed out what I thought should have been obvious to those in positions of leadership. The population was in a panic. Americans were desperate for sensible policymakers who had the courage to ignore the fear and rely on the facts. Leaders must examine accumulated data—and there was quite a bit of it by then from all over the world—rather than emphasizing hypothetical projections of models, combine that empirical evidence with fundamental principles of biology established for decades, and then thoughtfully restore the country to full function.

I listed five key facts being ignored by those calling for continuing the total lockdown, including that the overwhelming majority of people do not have any significant risk of dying from COVID-19; that we had a clearly defined population at high risk who could be protected with targeted measures; and that people were dying, as other medical care was not getting done due to the shutdowns and fear of entering a medical facility.

Instead I advocated a more focused protection model that would entail increasing protection of the elderly, who were dying at high rates because they were not being protected by the lockdowns, while allowing younger, healthy people with an extremely low risk to function, so that the harms of the lockdown would end. I specifically urged "to institute a more focused strategy, like some outlined in the first place: strictly protect the known vulnerable, self-isolate the mildly sick, and open most workplaces and small businesses with some prudent large-group precautions." This would save lives, prevent overcrowding of hospitals, and limit the enormous harms compounded by continued isolation. I urgently called for policymakers to stop underemphasizing empirical evidence while they instead doubled down on hypothetical models.

That publication went viral. The public clearly responded to logic and common sense. I cited extensive data in simple terms and also explained long-established principles of biology. Average people understood facts when presented clearly, but these straightforward facts had been glaringly absent from public discussion. One might conclude that "experts" didn't trust average Americans to comprehend facts, but that couldn't be the whole story. Could it be that they were simply incompetent, that they did not know or understand or didn't bother to critically question the data?

Perhaps the newly found fame of public health officials and modelers provided an incentive too irresistible to back down on their claims. Perhaps their interpretations were influenced by a financial incentive—for instance, many derived research dollars from those most influential in allocating those funds or even direct financial benefit from board positions with vaccine and drug companies. Or perhaps their motivations were driven by political rage against a president they despised and desperately wanted to bring down, even if it took a horrendous crisis to do it. One thing was clear to me—regardless of their motivations, most of the so-called experts advocating lockdowns had proved themselves to be pseudoscientists, today's "Flat Earthers" propagating terribly harmful misinformation.

My piece in *The Hill* was ultimately shared over a million times and read by tens of millions throughout the world. It was reprinted in foreign media outlets. National network television news shows, syndicated radio programs, and dozens of regional media outlets started to interview me.

Martha MacCallum highlighted the publication to a large national audience on her nightly Fox News show. She spoke for millions of ordinary Americans when she asked me something no one before had explained: "So, you say that that most people in this country are not in danger of dying from COVID-19. Explain."

I answered with data—as I always did, citing statistics that were not articulated by those in charge of communicating with the American people, those on the podium with the president of the United States.

> "These are some of the key facts that we've learned. Point number one is that the overwhelming majority of people do not have any significant risk of dying. This is showing all over the world. And in fact, what induced the panic was this overestimation of what's called the fatality rate of the infection by the World Health Organization. But in reality, that's a fraction. So, if you take the number of people who are going to die and you divide it by the people who are infected, they got three to five percent of people, which is very high.

> "But now we know from data all over the world, including the US, that a massive number of people have the virus that were either asymptomatic. In fact, 50 percent of people that are infected have zero symptoms.

> "And then another large percentage have nothing really significant that demands any medical care and certainly not hospitalization. So, when you look at the newer data that has come out, the estimates are that the fatality rate is very low, maybe 0.1 percent…it's not known exactly. But these are estimates."

My point was that a massive number of infected people go undetected—as Bhattacharya's and other data had already shown. The WHO overstatement of the fatality rate was based on the "case fatality rate," i.e., only those who were sick enough to seek medical attention, rather than the "infection fatality rate," i.e., of all those who had the infection, whether sick or not. This was much more than an esoteric technicality. The hysteria was related to distortions of that very concept that confused the public about the death risk from SARS2. One was the grossly misleading comparison of the infection fatality ratio (IFR) of the flu, under 0.1 percent, with the case fatality rate (CFR) of this virus, said to be 3.4 percent, but more than tenfold higher than its IFR. The second damaging error was the false implication that the overall risk was similar for everyone. The inescapable yet ignored fact was the thousandfold difference in risk between elderly and the young: this coronavirus was less risky to children than seasonal influenza and only of high risk to the elderly and infirm.

Then I noted with simple facts what was already proven, all over the world, but was never emphasized by the faces of public health—namely, the significant difference in risk between the elderly, particularly those with underlying illnesses, and everyone else:

> And we also know that when you take the people are going to die. This is New York data: two-thirds of people are over 70. 95 percent of people are over 50. If you're young and healthy, you have essentially zero, near zero chance of dying. And then the last part of who is at risk to die are when you look at the hotbed in the U.S., New York City. It's something like 99.2 percent today's data of all those investigated for underlying conditions. 99.2 percent had some underlying condition.

MacCallum delved further: "And what are the most prevalent among those (risk factors)?" I stated the facts for the public, as they were already widely recognized:

> If you take away age, the number one underlying condition is obesity and diabetes.... Although it's not clear how [quantifiably] impactful each one of these is, there's not a lot of good data on these. But

other diseases [too] like kidney disease, congestive heart failure.

I then restated the bottom line, again with data, because viewers wanted, deserved, and needed to know the facts:

If you're young and otherwise healthy, you have essentially zero risk of dying.... If you're under 18 in New York, you make up 0.6 percent of the hospitalizations. And if you're over 60 you make up two-thirds. So, there is a very significant targeted population here. We need to protect them—that doesn't need total isolation [of everyone].

At that moment, and during the interviews that followed, I silently questioned the motivation of public health officials and medical scientists at our universities who were frankly denying the science, as well as an irresponsible media who were sensationalizing and perpetuating the false narratives without any balancing perspective.

Over the next thirty days I submitted to fifty interviews and podcasts. There was nothing in my words that should have been controversial. But it was shocking to many, because I was countering the widely held but false narrative that had gripped the nation, indeed the world.

That false story—that this coronavirus was far more deadly than the flu by several orders of magnitude; that everyone is at high risk to die; that no one has any immune protection, because it is entirely new; that everyone was spreading the virus widely; that locking down and isolating everyone was urgently needed; and that the only protection would be from a vaccine, and that was years away—was an epic failure of both public health officials and the media, one that incited extraordinarily harmful, tragically misguided policies.

It became clear that this struck a chord in people. They were thirsty for a logical presentation of what was happening. They wanted the evidence and straightforward data, not hyperbole and theoretical models; they wanted calm leadership, not panic. I began to receive hundreds and then thousands of emails from all over the United States and around the world. Almost all were positive. People were desperate and highly emotional, encouraging me to continue speaking out.

I also received dozens, hundreds, of emails from epidemiologists, medical scientists, doctors, biostatisticians—agreeing with me, sending me their own research, and sadly telling me they personally were afraid to speak out, but that I should keep going, keep citing the facts. I received pleas from parents, from teachers, from school board members begging me not to give up, to stay visible, and keep telling the truth.

But from a few colleagues at Stanford University, I received very different reactions. One psychiatry professor at Stanford School of Medicine, who lives on my block, warned me that "right wing media were using me." I was stunned. At the time, I was still naively assuming that, like me, medical scientists would care about the data and nothing else. OK, I thought, most Stanford professors were understandably ignorant of the data. They hadn't studied it in depth, apparently. And, true, they were not in the field of health policy, my field of expertise. But to admonish me because my analysis and policy views were aired on media they considered unacceptable? I was totally disgusted. First, I never solicited a single interview—for every interview, the media contacted me. Martha MacCallum of Fox News asked, and I accepted. CNN? They never requested an interview back then. Second, I never considered declining or accepting an interview invitation due to the political slant of the media outlet. I was contacted because of my research and expertise, and I agreed to appear so people could understand the emergency at hand. Anyway, this was data, facts, critical information. The country was in the midst of the biggest health care crisis in a century—but the conservative slant of the media broadcasting my policy views was the concern of Stanford medical school professors?

Like my neighbor, in a community where 95 percent of political donations went to Democrats, some apparently couldn't get over their rage against President Trump and anything that might divert from their mission of bringing him down. Perhaps that was their reason for attacking the research coming from exceptional scientists like Ioannidis, Bhattacharya, and others. Was it possible that otherwise smart people, people normally able to engage in critical thinking, people skilled at examining data, had succumbed to an unconscious—or even conscious—desire for this negative fear-inducing story to continue during the election season? At the time I discarded the thought. In retrospect, however, that reproach by my neighbor was a harbinger of things to come.

* * * * *

In a series of publications, radio and television interviews, and podcasts I continued to push for increased protections for those most at risk, particularly the elderly, who were dying by the tens of thousands because the chosen policies were failing to protect them. I emphasized the science, and it showed that children were at extremely low risk for serious illness or death, that children were not significant spreaders of the infection, and that the overwhelming majority of people had asymptomatic or relatively mild disease from this infection.

At that time, New York City was the world's hotbed for COVID, when they had 130,000 cases and more than one-third of all US deaths. Of all fatal cases in New York, two-thirds were patients over seventy years of age, and more than 95 percent were over fifty. For people with COVID under eighteen years old, the rate of death was *zero per 100,000*. Of the first 6,570 COVID-19 deaths in NYC fully investigated for health status, 6,520, or 99.2 percent, had an underlying illness. It was clear that if you do not already have an underlying chronic condition, your chances of dying are small, *regardless of age.*

It wasn't just the data on deaths that was invisible in the media coverage. In New York, even for people ages sixty-five to seventy-four, only 1.7 percent were hospitalized. Half of all people testing positive for infection have no symptoms at all. The vast majority of younger, otherwise healthy people do not need significant medical care if they catch this infection. And young adults and children in normal health have almost no risk of any serious illness from COVID-19.

At the same time, I stressed that the appropriate goal of public health policy is to minimize all harms, not simply to stop COVID-19 at all costs. Treatments, including emergency care, for the most serious illnesses were also missed. Half of cancer patients deferred their chemotherapy. An estimated 80 percent of brain surgery cases were skipped. Up to half of acute stroke and heart attack patients missed their only chances for treatment, some dying and many now facing permanent disability. Most cancer screenings were skipped. Meanwhile there was tremendous harm from closing schools, shuttering businesses, and confining people to their homes—and all these harms were worse for lower-income families. All this was already shown by the data. Why in the world was it being ignored, literally denied, by the experts we were relying on to guide our nation?

That May, I was asked to testify before the Senate Committee on Homeland Security. I reviewed the latest data, but my purpose was to instill some perspective on policy. I wrote in my statement, "We now have an even greater urgency, due to the severe and single-minded policies already implemented. Treating Covid-19 'at all costs' is severely restricting other medical care and instilling fear in the public, creating a massive health disaster, in addition to severe economic harms that could generate a world poverty crisis with almost incalculable consequences."

I introduced the senators to critical background data that all policymakers should have been communicating to the public at the time:

> Reassuring the public about re-entry requires repeating the facts—what we know—about the threat and who it targets. By now, multiple studies from Europe, Japan, and the US all suggest that the overall fatality rate is far lower than early estimates, perhaps below 0.1 to 0.4%, i.e., ten to forty times lower than estimates that motivated extreme

isolation. And we also now know who to protect, because this disease—by the evidence—is not equally dangerous across the population. In Detroit's Oakland County, 75 percent of deaths were in those over 70; 91 percent were in people over 60, similar to what was noted in New York. And younger, healthier people have virtually zero risk of death and little risk of serious disease—as I have noted before, under one percent of New York City's hospitalizations have been patients under 18 years of age, and less than one percent of deaths at any age are in the absence of underlying conditions.

I continued with specific recommendations for a more effective, targeted strategy. I outlined in blunt terms that the implemented lockdowns were failing. I listed several specific ways to increase mitigation, to augment the protection of the elderly and other high-risk individuals, and to safely reopen society.

First, I told the Senate, let's finally focus on protecting the most vulnerable—that means nursing home patients. By then, more than a third of all deaths in the US, more than half in some states, were in nursing homes, where they already live under controlled access. We should strictly require testing and protective masks for all who entered, I urged. I warned that no COVID-19-positive patient should resume residence there until definitively cleared by testing. I also told them to reinforce that those with mild symptoms of the illness should strictly self-isolate for two weeks, and wear protective masks when others in their homes enter the same room.

But the senators mostly needed to understand the harms of the shutdowns. I stressed opening all K-12 schools, with standards for protecting elderly and other at-risk family members or friends, including teachers in higher-risk groups. If under eighteen and in good health, you have nearly no risk of any serious illness from COVID-19. Why was that ignored?

We needed to open most businesses, including restaurants and offices, but require new standards for hygiene. Public transportation, the lifeblood of much of the workforce in cities, should resume with new standards of cleanliness. Given the state of our fearful public, it seemed likely that most people would wear masks, even if they weren't required.

And I added what should have been obvious: parks and beaches should open with considered limits on large group gatherings. They knew it, but it had to be said on the record: "There is no scientific reason to insist that people remain indoors."

I concluded my testimony with the following summary on minimizing all health harms and saving all lives:

> Targeted protection for the known vulnerable, standards and commonsense recommendations for individuals and businesses, and prioritized testing form the basis of an urgently needed, strategic re-entry plan that would save lives, prevent overcrowding of hospitals, and limit the enormous harms compounded by continued total isolation.

All these recommendations were directly based on and consistent with scientific data. My recommendations also contrasted with the policies in place throughout the country, policies that bizarrely failed to consider all health harms from both the infection and the policies themselves. At that same committee hearing, John Ioannidis and David Katz, the author of an earlier piece in the *New York Times* on focused protection, spoke in very similar terms.

Simultaneously, it struck me that the massive, undeniable damage to businesses, jobs, and the economy was going to be devastating. Entire sectors would be wiped out, like travel and hospitality, and all the businesses directly and indirectly tied to them. It was not the corporations and large companies that would suffer. It was the workers, the small businesses and their employees, the waiters, the janitors, the delivery drivers and shippers, the cooks. It was the entire working class, the low-income families, the single-parent mothers and fathers. Entire communities would be devastated.

It wasn't just inside the United States, either. For many counties, international travel and business represented the mainstay of their economies. Over a hundred million people worldwide would be swept into abject poverty. Entire countries dependent on the West's demand, like Bangladesh's dependence on garment manufacturing, would be wiped out. Meanwhile I watched with disgust the disgraceful comments of elites broadcasting from their multimillion-dollar estates as they commiserated with their entertainment friends about how "we're all doing our share" and complained about their trivial inconveniences.

A false dichotomy had been set up to the effect that the desire to end the lockdown was somehow choosing money over lives. This blatant disregard for decades of economic literature documenting that income and jobs correlate directly to lives and health could only be explained in one way. The public discussion was poisoned, filtered by an irresponsible press plainly motivated by a political agenda. The president had said many times that he wanted to open the economy, that "the cure couldn't be worse than the problem." Once again, there was a noticeable absence of urgently needed analysis from those expected to help. I asked myself, sitting on a university campus filled with highly regarded economics professors, "Where are the economists?"

Eventually I found one, or should I say one found me. During May, I was contacted by John Birge, an economist at the University of Chicago Booth School of Business. He and some of his colleagues—Ralph Keeney, professor emeritus at Duke University and at the University of Southern California; and Alex Lipton, a brilliant mathematician, quantitative analyst, and computer scientist—had noticed my work and were interested in collaborating on a piece about the economic devastation from the lockdowns. We published our article in late May in *The Hill*. In doing so, we were among the first to quantify the lives lost from the lockdown and compare that to the losses from the virus.

To ensure that we were very conservative in our estimates, we limited ourselves to published actuarial data about life-years lost from two consequences of the lockdowns—missed health care and lost jobs. We restricted our study to a small set of health care data (stroke, chemotherapy, new cancer cases, transplants, and certain childhood vaccinations). The second category tallied life-years lost, the economist's statistic that accounted for age of death from unemployment alone. We wrote, "Considering only the losses of life from missed health care and unemployment due solely to the lockdown policy, we conservatively estimate that the national lockdown is responsible for at least 700,000 lost years of life every month, or about 1.5 million so far—already far surpassing the COVID-19 total."

Our conclusion stated an undeniable truth that had not been emphasized to the public, despite months of lockdowns: "The belated acknowledgment by policy leaders of irreparable harms from the lockdown is not nearly enough. They need to emphatically and widely inform the public of these serious consequences and reassure them of their concern for all human life by strongly articulating the rationale for reopening society."

*　*　*　*　*

I was particularly beside myself about one specific part of the lockdowns—school closures. The most obvious denial of science, the most egregious and inexplicable failure of policy leadership in our country, was indefinitely closing schools. For weeks, I had been highlighting data showing the extremely low risk to children arising from the virus. I cited study after study documenting that while kids could get infected, and while there were exceptions, they had nearly zero risk for death. Their risk for hospitalization was also extremely low. I specifically pointed out CDC data on the first 60,000 deaths; only 12 had been in children. I focused on New York City, at the time the US epicenter of COVID. In NYC data at the end of May, of the 15,756 deaths that had occurred, only 8 (0.05 percent) were less than eighteen years old; only one child had no underlying condition.

I specifically cited the May 2020 *JAMA* review of North American pediatric hospitals. That study flatly stated: "Our data indicate that children are at far greater risk of critical illness from influenza than from COVID-19." For children, COVID was far less serious than in adults, even less serious than the common flu.

By all logic, I repeatedly said, "If we are going to close schools for this, then we would need to close schools for influenza, too— every year for the flu season, have everyone wear masks during flu season, have every child separated by six feet during flu season." Of course that had never been recommended, despite the fact that hundreds of children died annually from the flu, a far higher percentage than from COVID, according to CDC, and children were a significant source of transmitted influenza, a disease that killed tens of thousands of high-risk elderly every year.

Teacher unions were instrumental in paralyzing parents with fear by lying about the danger in schools. And beyond the extremely low risk to kids, the vast majority of teachers themselves are not even in the high-risk group. I pointed out the facts—that public K-12 teachers are a young profession, with a median forty-one years of age. A full 92 percent are under sixty.

The bottom line was this: America was uniquely hysterical in its disregard of actual data on schools and children, more off the rails than almost anywhere in the world. I remember later asking Kayleigh McEnany, the president's press secretary, "What kind of country sacrifices its children out of fear for adults?" To me, this was a sin, a total breakdown of the moral contract between a civilization and its children. I asked myself, "Where are the teachers? Where are the pediatricians and child psychologists? And where are the parents?"

On June 1, I published a piece on reopening schools in *The Hill* with my colleague Paul Peterson. Dr. Peterson is an education policy scholar and director of the Program on Education Policy and Governance at Harvard University. In late May, Peterson had interviewed me on his *Education Next* podcast about school closures that had been implemented that spring, and in our coauthored piece, we countered the outrageous lie being perpetrated by the teacher unions that schools somehow represented a danger. We cited data from the CDC stating: "[O]f the first 68,998 U.S. deaths from

COVID-19, only 12 have been in children under age 14—less than 0.02 percent. Nor is coronavirus killing teenagers. At last count, the fatality total among children under 18 without an underlying condition is one; only ten of the 16,469 confirmed coronavirus deaths in New York City were among those under the age of 18."

We noted that similar data had been compiled in several countries in Europe. And we compared it to the far higher danger to kids from flu, COVID-19 fatalities numbered just twelve, but several hundreds of children in the United States died from seasonal influenza in 2017–18, according to CDC estimates. We also showed what was already proven back in May 2020: "As is shown across the world, including Switzerland, Canada, the Netherlands, France, Iceland, the UK, Australia and now Ireland, children seldom if ever transmit the disease to adults, even to their parents."

Later, the Swedish Public Health Agency reported that throughout the 2020 spring wave, Sweden kept daycare and schools open for every one of its 1.8 million children aged between one and sixteen. All their schools were open without subjecting them to testing, masks, physical barriers, or social distancing. The results? Exactly zero COVID deaths in kids, while Sweden's teachers had a COVID risk similar to the average of other professions. Schools were not high-risk settings.

Peterson and I listed only some of the problems with school closures, because none of the spokesmen in public health leadership pointed out these extraordinary harms to the public. Instead, most public health officials stressed the exceptional rarities of multisystem inflammatory disorder, an extremely rare and treatable consequence, statements that only exposed their lack of clinical perspective that is crucial in understanding the illness.

We also wrote that online education was a failure, a fact that was only validated further as more data came in. For example, we reported that in Boston, only half of students were showing up for online instruction on any given day, and 20 percent had never logged on to the designated website. And that failure was especially impacting low-income kids: "Many lack WIFI, computer tablets, software and other paraphernalia of the affluent. Nor are they as likely to have access to equivalent mentors at home as those with better educated parents. Robin Lake at the Center for Reinventing Public Education says that 'elementary students [in urban districts] may have lost 30 percent of their reading skills.'"

Meanwhile serious health harms to kids, who had no significant risk from the illness itself, were being created by school closures. The data had already shown that more than half of America's children were not receiving needed vaccinations. "Further," we noted, "schools are the place where many learn that they need glasses or a hearing aid, or, if seriously ill, are guided by the school nurse to the doctor's office for prompt medical attention."

What parent or teacher didn't fully understand that children were being denied "opportunities for social and emotional development that come with play, exercise, sports and socialization"? Economically as well, we pointed out that a lasting loss in lifetime earnings would occur. Meanwhile, suicide rates among the young were already on the rise. We concluded: "Risks from COVID-19 are too minimal to sacrifice the educational, social, emotional and physical well-being—to say nothing of the very health—of our young people."

Only later did data pour in on the approximately 300,000 unreported child abuse cases from those spring closures alone—missed because schools are the number one agency where such abuse is noted. Only later, in July, would the CDC report that one in four young people aged eighteen to twenty-four had contemplated suicide. Only later would staggering failure rates be noted—a 40–70 percent rise in failing grades during online distance learning in Virginia, for instance. And only later would the more damaging impacts come out, like a tripling of self-harm in teenagers requiring doctor visits, an explosion of anxiety and depression, a massive weight gain averaging twenty-eight pounds in more than half of college-aged kids during the lockdowns, and a morbid fear of all social interaction by the end of the year.

Meanwhile, in the US, lockdown proponents and teacher unions pushed for maintaining school closures. That policy, advocated by the political class, exposed another total failure of perspective by the affluent on how the lockdowns harmed working-class families. Keeping schools closed would severely limit the ability of parents to work. A whopping 79 percent of single-mother families and 88 percent of single-father families with kids six to seventeen have jobs. How would they be able to work if their kids were out of school?

These and my other written pieces—filled with statistics and scientific references—with millions of readers were featured on national and international news, and some were reprinted in full throughout the world. I conducted almost a hundred interviews in the late spring to early summer on television, radio, podcasts, and other digital media. In every interview, I cited data and quoted specific publications from scientific journals. The draconian lockdowns, the strangely unscientific mandates on behavior that either had no basis in evidence or were directly counter to scientific data, continued.

The narrow, poorly thought out, unscientific lockdown policy advocated by the president's leading experts stunned me. Ignoring the enormous harms of the lockdowns, I thought, was profoundly immoral behavior on the part of those in charge of the nation's health policy. The fundamental obligation of anyone in public health leadership included considering all the potential harms of a policy, not simply trying to stop an infection regardless of other social costs. Meanwhile people kept dying, including the known high-risk elderly who should have been protected from the outset.

At times, it became difficult to suppress my frustration in interviews. These points were fairly simple, yet so many were denying them, and the policies were implemented almost everywhere. Why didn't facts matter?

* * * * *

At this point I began having informal conversations with state and federal government officials. I was encouraged by their intellectual curiosity and their concern to understand the data, rather than to blindly accept what they were told. Most were asking me to explain my rationale for how to proceed. One official stood out, though.

As I was sitting at my desk overflowing with papers and notes and going through about thirty websites that I kept open, Florida Governor Ron DeSantis called me. He briefly introduced himself and asked me a series of specific questions about the pandemic. But the unique and impressive nature of the call was that this governor had an extraordinarily high level of familiarity with the data—and not simply the data in Florida. He had at his fingertips all the key statistics and trends from the rest of the country, as well as Europe and elsewhere. DeSantis kept posing his interpretations and asking if he was correct. He was virtually always right. Moreover, he displayed an amazingly sophisticated grasp of the scientific literature—far better than the "credentialed experts" appearing on cable TV.

Given that Florida was particularly vulnerable due to its high concentration of elderly, he was focused on how to protect them. The governor was shocked at the New York governor's directive plainly ordering that COVID-positive patients discharged from hospitals could not be prevented from returning to nursing homes ("No resident shall be denied re-admission or admission to the [nursing home] solely based on a confirmed or suspected diagnosis of COVID-19"). The *Wall Street Journal* reported this at the end of March, and I was stunned. I told DeSantis that the policy was totally inexplicable, grossly incompetent, and in my opinion a complete disqualifier for anyone in a leadership position.

Everyone in medicine and public health knew that a nursing home was a tinderbox of risk. Deadly infection outbreaks were already well documented in nursing homes, including past influenza outbreaks. For example, in California's 2017–2018 flu season, 88 percent of outbreaks occurred in nursing homes and assisted-living facilities. These elderly residents were the most vulnerable of all, more than obvious hazards from their frailty and group indoor-living situations as well as their frequent encounters with staff from the community.

I told Governor DeSantis that such a policy was beyond negligent; he agreed. And New York was not the only state leadership that placed those people into nursing homes—that list included Pennsylvania, New Jersey, and Michigan. I told DeSantis that in my opinion this policy would be—and likely already was—responsible for killing nursing home residents. We both had ideas for increasing protections in nursing homes.

Beyond his remarkable attention to detail, another characteristic of my conversations with the governor was what I would call his healthy degree of skepticism, which I believe is essential to arrive at the truth. There was already an established narrative. But if one was to be sure of its conclusions, it was necessary to question them. DeSantis expressed great concern about the harms of missed medical care, the enormous damage to kids from school closures, the impact of isolation on the elderly, and the damage to working families from societal shutdowns. We would intermittently touch base over the rest of the summer about the trends, their implications, and policies to protect at-risk citizens.

Throughout the spring and summer of 2020, I relentlessly consumed the scientific literature on the virus, immunity and susceptibility, risk factors for serious illness, and a host of other issues. Every detail and update on websites of the CDC, the *New York Times*, and other databases, and throughout Europe was important. Twitter, with all its obvious flaws, was an additional way to find up-to-the minute links to publications and interviews. I developed regular interaction with a number of dedicated people interested in analyzing data about the pandemic. I was also receiving a continual stream of publications and updates on the scientific literature, as well as the source data on trends of cases, hospitalizations, and deaths. It became a part of my routine to speak with a number of individuals who were feeding me detailed, corrected data that was embedded deep beneath the inadequate journalistic depictions.

I read publications and listened to interviews from many of the world's leading authorities on epidemiology, virology, and infectious diseases. Dozens of outstanding scientists were publishing vital data, often evading attempts to silence research by using expedited, pre-formal-acceptance digital versions. In addition to John Ioannidis and Jay Bhattacharya, both of whom continued to publish extremely important and highly impactful studies, Dr. Sunetra Gupta, a brilliant Oxford University scientist and one of the world's most accomplished epidemiologists, was bravely detailing the flawed assumptions of the original models. She, too, stated without fear that this obsession with testing and "cases" as defined by those tests was misguided, severely harmful, and scientifically inappropriate. Drs. Carl Heneghan and Tom Jefferson, exceptional scientists at Oxford's Centre for Evidence-Based Medicine, were also pointing out valuable science about masks, testing, and other critical issues in the face of a prevailing but unscientific backlash.

Meanwhile, labs from all over the world were publishing important studies about related viruses. I had not yet heard of Dr. Martin Kulldorff, professor of medicine at Harvard Medical School, another renowned epidemiologist. Only months later, in September, did I become aware that he had been censored in the United States, because he was writing against the school lockdowns. In August 2020, his first US media op-ed was finally published by CNN…but only in their CNN-Espanol edition. (CNN-English wasn't interested, according to Martin, so he wrote it in Spanish to get it published.)

Several times a week, I went over the key data and new research separately with Drs. Ioannidis and Bhattacharya. Nearly every conversation began with me being agitated about the profoundly off-base words of scientists all over the world. I could not understand the frank denial of fundamental biology and disregard for the massive body of evidence on the pandemic risks, on the immune response, and on the lack of efficacy of masks that had swiftly accumulated. I was astounded by the Kafkaesque lack of logic that had consumed the pandemic narrative. I kept asking, "Where are the scientists?" Ioannidis reminded me of the low level of scholarship that was rampant in medical research, a fact he exposed in his heavily cited 2005 essay entitled, "Why Most Published Research Findings Are False." And nearly every conversation ended the same way. They never let me give up, they never stopped encouraging me, and they always did their best, with good humor, to calm me down by saying over and over again: "Scott, don't worry. The truth will prevail."

The stream of emails from scientists, doctors, and researchers increased to the point where I couldn't come close to responding. I was staggered by the number of academicians who told me they were afraid to speak out or were having a difficult time getting their research published. Most of that research was scientifically and methodologically solid, but because it went against the prevailing narrative, it was rejected. This unimaginable suppression of research by scientific journals was frightening. How in the world would the truth be discovered, if the very research that led to it was censored? Since when was it OK for scientists and academics to demonize researchers who simply put forth their interpretation of data?

My inbox was also filling up with emails from increasingly desperate parents, senior citizens, and people from all walks of life throughout the US and other countries. Most of them thanked me for speaking up and appealing to common sense. Those emails from ordinary Americans frankly changed my mindset, from one of frustration and bewilderment to one of a larger purpose. These everyday people depended on someone knowledgeable to give voice to what they, deep down, understood: that although the virus was serious and some people were at high risk, the lockdowns were a massive mistake, a hugely destructive policy, an irrational overimposition on the public that needed to stop.

By summer of 2020, the public was extremely fragile due to the ongoing pandemic and its draconian management. Almost two hundred thousand Americans had died, severe lockdowns were in place, and no end was in sight. The fear was exacerbated by improper public health leadership and an irresponsible, politicized media. A running dashboard of cases occupied the broadcasts 24/7. Sensationalized stories about every new consequence, no matter how rare, were at the top of the hour on the news. A National Bureau of Economic Research (NBER) study from Dartmouth and Brown later proved the extremely negative bias of American media—a true outlier to the world's English-speaking news on COVID-19. From January through July 2020, 91 percent of stories by US major media outlets were negative in tone versus 54 percent for major news sources outside the US. On nearly every important issue—from the safety of opening schools to the potential arrival of a vaccine—America's news outlets were the world's outlier: uniquely negative, delaying and omitting positive news while amplifying and even stressing negative information. The NBER study reported that stories of increasing COVID cases outnumbered stories of decreasing cases by a factor of 5.5 even when new cases were declining. Statistics were presented in the most fear-invoking way, and any uncertainty was highlighted, regardless of its relative lack of clinical importance.

It was undeniable that this was intentional, regardless of the true motive. But when considered along with the overt hostility in the press toward Donald Trump, it was difficult to believe that the negative presentation was not at least in part politically motivated, especially then, just a few months ahead of the 2020 election.

In addition to their unrelenting emphasis on negative news, many media outlets seemed to be pushing the narrative that this president "didn't listen to the science." After all, embarrassing conflicts between the president and his media-friendly advisor, Dr. Fauci, had become highly visible and were frequently featured on cable news shows. Fauci was advising continued lockdowns, while the president was calling for reopening of schools and businesses. The president had extolled the promise of various experimental drug treatments, while Fauci had insisted that vaccines were the only way out of the pandemic.

Fauci was inconsistent about mask efficacy, first stating that they were not effective and then changing completely—even though Oxford University's Centre for Evidence-Based Medicine, the CDC, and a body of literature and evidence in this pandemic showed that population masks were not effective in stopping the spread of the infection. He also insisted that the coronavirus was virtually proven to be natural and confidently assured us that it had originated from a market in Wuhan, while the president was suggesting the virus probably leaked from China's virus research laboratory just down the road that worked on the same family of viruses.

I personally couldn't have cared less about any conflicts between Fauci and President Trump—that seemed like political drama played up by the media. The problem was that such conflicts added to the uncertainty of the viewing public, undermining the public's trust in what was being done to manage the pandemic. I never thought in detail about the origin of the virus or the controversies about the drug treatments or the erratic press conference remarks I had seen on TV. The far bigger problem was my focus: the advice coming out of the Task Force was inflicting massive damage, especially to children, working families, and the poor—all while failing to save the elderly. The positions of these public health officials were in conflict with emerging research and empirical evidence that their policies were failing. The lockdown advocates, led by Drs. Fauci and Birx, were disregarding concerns about total health in pushing unprecedented, severe societal lockdowns to stop COVID-19 at all costs, policies implemented by states that inflicted incalculable damage and death.

Even beyond the flawed policies and seeming lack of concern by policymakers about their consequences, the public fear itself was a very important problem, one that had to be addressed. Almost all of the public health officials appearing in the media seemed to be adding to the fear and confusion. I thought Dr. Fauci could have done better to assure the nation about what we already knew to be true. By explaining what the data had already shown and what was reasonable to infer from decades of knowledge, he could have removed some of the uncertainty, reduced the fear, and helped calm the nation. More facts were available, important details, yet they remained almost invisible.

On May 18, 2020, I published another widely read piece in *The Hill*. The purpose was to educate the public and hopefully impact the way people thought about the pandemic. The more facts that were put forward, I believed, the less fear and anxiety there would be.

After arguing that the public had not been given key messages critical to alleviating fear and guiding a safe reopening of society, I listed specific failures in leadership, including:

- "A failure to educate the public that the overall fatality rate is not only far lower than previously thought but is extremely low in almost everyone other than the elderly."

- "A failure to clarify to parents the truth about the extremely low risk to children, and that has accompanied a gross failure to offer a rational medical perspective regarding schools reopening."

- "Public statements by scientists and the media that sensationalize…extremely rare instances are particularly harmful, because they instill undue fear and provoke extraordinarily harmful, misguided policies from people who lack a medical perspective."

Finally, I identified "the real failure": "Public policy must never be one-dimensional. It can never be foisted on people without careful consideration of its consequences, including the harms from the well-intentioned attempt to solve the initial problem…. It's time to stop the cycle of becoming frantic as we see what are totally expected changes in hypothetical projections. Instead, let's use empirical evidence and established medical science."

What really threw me was that the editor of *The Hill* convinced me to soften the title of my essay. I listened in astonishment as he advised me that it would have been made invisible on Google and Facebook if I maintained my submitted title, "What Dr. Fauci Failed to Say," which I thought was a straightforward, rather bland headline. After more than an hour of conversation, we agreed on the less critical wording, "Adding to Dr. Fauci's Diagnosis." I was surprised that during a national crisis, when all voices and perspectives were desperately needed, the sensitivity was focused on not offending Google and Facebook. It was my awakening to the censorship of the tech giants that controlled access to information. In retrospect, that conversation also indicated the cowardice of many in the media. That, too, was a harbinger of more storms to come—the crime to avoid, the most unforgivable offense of all to many people, was simply disagreeing with Dr. Fauci.

At the end of that hectic and at times dispiriting spring and early summer, I received a call from my mother-in-law. She told me that Kayleigh McEnany, the White House press secretary, was quoting me in press conferences, citing my statistics on children, on why schools should open. I was surprised, but I took it as a cause for some optimism. Could it be that facts and logic might prevail over the series of obsessions and misconceptions that had taken hold? My mother-in-law predicted, "Scott, you are going to Washington." I laughed and assured her that was not happening.

Throughout those months, every single discussion at our family dinner table consisted of me ranting about the data, explaining its implications, and even reviewing the latest science publications. Several times a day, I was telling them, "The country is off the rails," something they got tired of hearing. I would show them my charts, illustrating flaws in logic and misconceptions that were continually stated in the media. My wife, always a critical thinker as well as a very tough audience, kept challenging me with questions. But she was more concerned that I was so visibly and publicly going against the dominant narrative in an increasingly contentious time. More than once she memorably warned: "I hope you're right."

CHAPTER 2
Off to Washington

It was the middle of July 2020. My day started the usual way—waking up at 6:00 a.m., making two cappuccinos, grabbing a piece of coffee cake, then heading upstairs to a bedroom that I had fashioned into an office during the pandemic. Prepared, I started my daily data review. I was determined to get to the bottom of the trends involving cases, testing, hospitalizations, and deaths.

Per usual, I closely evaluated several pieces of information. First, I looked at a series of "COVID dashboards" that featured data from selected countries, including the United States. I further examined data from every single state as well as several metropolitan areas. I also ran through the newest data from the CDC and several other health organizations. I then proceeded to comb through the latest peer-reviewed essays and other pertinent publications.

At that point, I was also having near-daily discussions about the existing evidence with top epidemiologists and infectious-disease scientists, including Stanford's Jay Bhattacharya and John Ioannidis. They both kept reassuring me that my interpretation of the data was accurate, and insisted that I persevere. We believed—and have since been proved right—that COVID-19 posed very little risk to the overwhelming majority of the population. So the focus should have been on protecting the known high-risk groups, instead of quarantining everyone. And all the efforts at stopping the cases by restricting everyone's movements, shutting down schools and businesses, and quarantining healthy people were failing to stop the known high-risk people, most notably the elderly, from dying.

Just as important, the lockdowns were destructive, inflicting great harm on society. In every conversation, John and Jay both sensed my own panic taking hold. "The truth will prevail," John repeatedly assured me. Jay encouraged me as well: "Keep it up, Scott, you're right! The tide is turning. I know it!" They were insistent on being optimistic, but I had my doubts. "I feel like I'm living in a Kafka novel!" I kept repeating at home and finally even said in some interviews. A lack of logic and common sense was already pervasive and crippling the country. The policies in place were wrong, yet the media unthinkingly touted them as if there were no alternative. And fear was everywhere. It had even paralyzed several members of my own family.

Around midday, my phone rang, interrupting my routine. It was John McEntee of the Personnel Office in the Executive Office of the President, who I later learned was one of President Trump's closest confidantes. In the coming months, we would talk frequently and candidly. We would agree on many key issues—especially who among the remarkable cast of West Wing characters was truly competent and who was dangerously inept.

In our initial call, McEntee asked a few questions about the trends and requested my perspective on managing the pandemic. He also offered his own guesses about the course ahead and thoughts on what should have been done, including the original shutdown. He wanted my reaction. The conversation then turned to an informal vetting.

"Have you engaged in any political activism?" he asked.

"No, I have not."

"Have you publicly aired any negative views, like on social media, hostile toward the president?"

"I have not."

McEntee also asked whom I had advised during the 2016 campaign. I listed several but told him I had declined to be named as a formal adviser to any particular candidate. He asked why I hadn't advised the president. "No one asked me to!" I responded. But I recounted my conversations with the Trump transition team, including whom I had recommended for heads of the FDA, CMS, HHS, and the other health care–related positions.

I apparently met his expectations, because he followed up with a slightly longer call a few days later.

"Would you be willing to fly out to Washington to meet the president?" he asked.

"Yes, of course," I quickly responded. "There's nothing more urgent than this crisis."

We decided that I would fly into Washington the following Sunday and visit the White House on Monday morning. There was no mention of anything beyond a single discussion.

After hanging up, I immediately spoke with my family and a couple of close friends. I felt there was no possible decision other than to accept. I was nervous but mostly relieved that I'd now have at least one chance to provide direct input at the highest levels.

My family and close friends, however, were very worried about the potential for a continued role after the first visit. They were concerned that I would be relentlessly attacked by the media, even in this patently nonpartisan role. They expected that I would be put out as disagreeing with Dr. Fauci and turned into a scapegoat for those who hated the president. They ultimately conceded it was essential to go, confident that I knew the data inside and out and, further, the policies that needed to be enacted. They recognized the country was "off the rails," a description I used too often at family dinners.

My family also understood that I would speak the truth—consequences be damned. I had never been afraid to voice my opinions. And no one would claim I was overly concerned about being delicate in that way. What's more, I had no ulterior motives. I was not auditioning. I didn't need that job or any other in government. I didn't care whether the White House would want me to remain in Washington. If they didn't like my message, I would be perfectly happy to keep delivering it from California. I was confident in my knowledge of the pandemic and in health policy, and that's all that mattered.

Some friends were emotional, almost ecstatic about the trip. They cheered that I would finally "right the ship"—that I would be "the anti-Fauci," or even replace him. I sternly corrected them. I had no intention of replacing anyone. I was simply going in order to offer my perspective. I also reminded them that this was unlikely to be anything beyond a short one-day trip.

*　*　*　*　*

During the five-hour flight from San Francisco to Washington, I felt uncertain about the actual point of the visit. I was confident that I would be direct about my thoughts. That part would be easy. I would finally have a chance to insert some common sense and a rational perspective into the national discussion surrounding the pandemic. In my mind, the entire narrative emanating from the highest-profile experts—and fawningly echoed by the media—was just plain wrong. And not just wrong, but extremely harmful.

Still, no one could deny that being associated with President Trump carried significant risk. I had watched the news every night and was repulsed by the media's vitriol. But if the administration asked that I stay on, perhaps I could advise him from a distance. My work, after all, had become fully virtual. I had been softly reprimanded for daring to work inside my closed office building at Stanford, though isolated in my personal office...in a totally deserted building...without any human contact.

I had decided to upgrade to business class, using frequent flyer miles earned from many trips as an invited speaker. Nonstop, in a flatbed. A good perk, I thought, even if this was going to be a waste of time.

After landing at Dulles Airport, we stood to exit the plane. I noticed a familiar face across the aisle, partially hidden under a mask, eyes darting around. At first, I couldn't place it. Then it hit me. It was Nancy Pelosi. I knew then that I was entering the heart of partisan politics, and I felt a pit in my stomach.

I hustled off the plane and through the terminal. As I left, I noticed a large security detail, presumably awaiting Pelosi. A Hoover colleague pulled up to the curb. We headed to the Willard Hotel, just one block east of the White House, to drop off my bags. We were then off to dinner.

The next morning, I entered the White House area through visitor security. I was brought to meet John McEntee at the Eisenhower Executive Office Building, known as the "EEOB," just across from the entrance to the West Wing. He and the others assembled in his office were excited to meet me. We were chatting when McEntee abruptly stopped.

"Did you get tested?" he asked.

"What do you mean?"

"You're going to meet the boss. You need a COVID test."

McEntee accompanied me to the ground floor of the EEOB, where I was tested. We then walked over to the West Wing to begin a series of appointments.

The morning and early afternoon were filled with one-on-one meetings with the president's inner circle: Mark Meadows, Jared Kushner, Stephen Miller, Kayleigh McEnany, Marc Short, Vice President Pence, and others less known to the public. Everyone was very welcoming, from the receptionists to those at the highest levels. I was stunned that everyone seemed to be intimately familiar with my statements and writings—and so enthusiastic that I had made the trip. All my discussions were very positive and focused on what I thought was happening with the pandemic. Some took notes as I spoke.

I spent more than an hour with Meadows over two separate meetings. Meadows was the President's chief of staff, one in a series of chiefs under this president. He was probably the bottom-line decider on the whole idea of any role I might have advising the president. This was a positive start—he demonstrated a solid handle on the data and the broader issues involved in the pandemic. McEnany showed me a list of my own talking points and quotes that she kept on her computer—that was a surprise that made me laugh. Miller was very sharp, intellectually engaged, and especially interested in getting feedback on his thoughts.

After my first meeting with Meadows, I bumped into the vice president as I was being escorted to my next appointment. He was warm and gracious. "Scott Atlas is here!" he boomed. "It's an honor to meet you, a great honor. Thank you so much for coming!" He said he was greatly looking forward to our meeting later in the day. I was taken aback. It was beyond any expectation to have the vice president of the United States offer such a kind welcome.

Then reality hit me. The vice president had some papers in his hands. With great pride, he excitedly showed me a printout that had just been handed to him. It was a very simple, frankly crude, chart documenting the increasing number of PCR tests administered by the day in the United States. "Congratulations!" I replied, feigning excitement. But inside, I realized something far more significant was being revealed.

The White House was looking at the simplest indicators—rudimentary numbers without detail, without context, without any concept of what actually mattered. The total number of tests was far from the critical part of the situation. We were already more than six months into the pandemic. What should have mattered was who was tested, when they were tested, what the testing revealed about contagiousness, and what positive testing meant in terms of action. That was my first "OMG" moment. This seemed like a naive reaction to political criticism, rather than what should have been in place by now, more than a half year later—a focused, well thought out plan of how to stop the destruction from the pandemic. I knew the country was really in deep trouble.

I continued on. I met with Kushner, alongside my friend John Rader, who worked closely with him. Kushner was very impressive, highly organized, and clearly "in charge" even though his job description was difficult to fully comprehend. He had no formal or informal presence on the Task Force. That said, he was the lead and most respected advisor and strategist to the president for pretty much everything, as far as I could tell. It was also far more than advising for many aspects of the executive branch's accomplishments—he was hands-on, working 24/7. He was also far more formal than everyone else.

"Hello, Doctor, thank you for coming," he opened.

"Hi, it's nice to meet you. And you can call me Scott."

"I will call you Doctor Atlas. You worked hard for that." And over the next four months, even though we met many times every week, Kushner always used that formal title.

During a discussion about the pandemic, someone strutted into the room with a printed-out draft of what would be a tweet from the president instructing that everyone should wear a mask. Kushner read it aloud, then turned to me.

"What do you think?" he asked.

In all honesty, I felt that the tweet's counsel was not rooted in scientific evidence. Rather, it seemed purely motivated by political considerations.

"Well, it conflicts with what the president has been saying about masks," I replied. I weighed stopping there but continued: "And it doesn't comport with the scientific data on general population masks, and it's not what the public health agencies wrote in their recommendations."

The person who brought in the tweet pushed back, reciting poll numbers about masks.

"Republicans also believe in masks for everyone," he pointed out, with irritation in his voice. Yep, I thought, this was going to be 100-percent political, a calculated decision to win votes. And to me, that should have been totally irrelevant.

"Well," I cautiously answered, "I would not want the president of the United States to state something that's scientifically incorrect, even it's the politically good thing to do. And he is already on record about masks, to wear them when appropriate, like in crowded places. Shouldn't he be consistent?"

My friend Rader, one of Jared's valued advisors, strongly agreed. Kushner paused, thinking it through, then modified the tweet on the spot to read, "Wear a mask when you cannot socially distance."

Emails about my itinerary were going back and forth between those escorting me, and I was intermittently updated on the whereabouts of my next meeting. I was informed that I had a lunch break.

After grabbing what was to become my standard lunch, a cappuccino and a chocolate chip cookie from the West Wing's "Navy Mess," I went to sit with Rader in his tiny office. I was then notified it was time to meet the president.

As we were heading up the stairs, I all of a sudden remembered my COVID test. I turned to Rader.

"What about my test results?"

He laughed. "If it were positive, you and every single person around would have known by now." As he would soon often do, he said with a big smile, "Good luck!"

CHAPTER 3
Welcome to the West Wing

Once upstairs, I introduced myself to the two receptionists sitting directly at the entrance to the Oval Office. The president was still finishing up a meeting, so I was led to the Cabinet Room. Most of it was occupied by a massive table, around which were placed approximately twenty chairs. Each back was individually labeled with an engraved plate, listing the name and appointment date of a cabinet secretary. I strolled around the room, checking out its historic paintings and sculptures. This was truly memorable.

Then the door swung open, and Stephen Miller walked in. We again chatted for about ten minutes. He left, and a few minutes later I was asked to enter the Oval Office.

I was struck by the room's size and grand feeling. A few people were stationed along the periphery, including Kushner, McEntee, and Mark Meadows. President Trump stood up from behind his desk with a big smile on his face and warmly welcomed me. He emanated positive energy.

"Here he is—the famous Dr. Atlas! Thank you for coming. It's a great honor to have you here!"

I smiled, thanked him for the opportunity to meet, and said something about the inability to shake hands due to concern for the virus. He gestured for me to have a seat directly in front of his desk, where there was a semicircle of four chairs spaced across the room. My focus was locked straight ahead, even though several pairs of eyes were on me from elsewhere in the room.

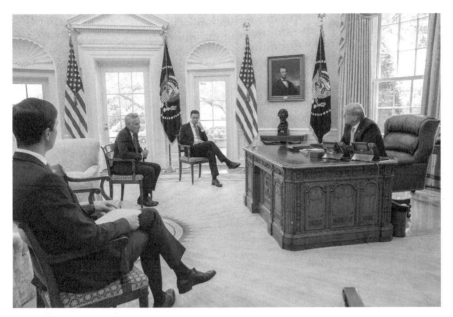

On my first visit to meet President Trump in the Oval Office, he and I talked about key issues in the pandemic while Jared Kushner (foreground) and Johnny McEntee watched. (*Credit: Official White House photographers*)

The president was not one to engage in small talk. He posed a rapid-fire series of questions about the pandemic. He asked what I thought lay ahead, about the initial shutdown ("You agree it was the right thing to do?"), the effectiveness of masks, the United States' performance relative to other countries, the continuing lockdowns, what should be done with schools, Sweden's strategy, testing people who were not sick, hydroxychloroquine, and a host of other questions. I went into some detail about harms from the lockdowns— facts about the missed cancer treatments, the skipped organ transplants, the cancers that were never diagnosed. I told him how the fear had caused people having heart attacks and strokes to avoid calling for an ambulance. I quickly cited some statistics about how school closures hurt children's learning and how hundreds of thousands of child abuse cases were never reported because they weren't detected by schools.

I was impressed that the president asked the right questions. He was very attentive, listening thoughtfully to every word and digesting the answers. My expectations were probably set too low owing to the constant criticism and ridicule of him by the media, but I was pleasantly surprised. It became obvious that he was upbeat about the interaction. I also sensed, even in this initial conversation, that he was frustrated—not just at how the country was still shut down, but that he had allowed it to happen, against his own intuition. At one point, he exclaimed with irritation in his voice, but to no one in particular, "Why the hell wasn't this guy here six months ago?" It was as if he understood that his closest advisors—several standing in that room—had somehow let him down. The meeting ended, and I walked out of the Oval Office and was joined by someone waiting to escort me to the rest of my meetings.

I spent some time with speechwriters. I went over suggestions about how to articulate what was happening, the important data, the need to be clear, and the need for the president himself to start speaking at the press conferences. Americans, I thought, were frightened, at least in part, due to uncertainty and a lack of information. I recommended what I had already told others, that the president himself present the data, with specifics, and illustrate to the American public that his administration was knowledgeable and engaged.

At this point, having been asked to provide specific ideas and words directly to the president's speechwriters, I began to realize that I had an incredible opportunity to help the country. Ordinary Americans were in full panic mode. In my mind, even simple common sense, rational discourse itself, was missing, and I couldn't help but think that was partly due to the political vitriol. But I was not political. I was a health policy expert, with a career steeped in data analysis. I could help translate the data for the president, so the public could deal with the fear and hopefully regain normal function. Teaching complex topics and simplifying data to arrive at the correct answer, using logic, was what I was known for in medicine over decades. I also understood how to articulate the massive harms from the lockdown policies—it had particularly frustrated me that the president was never able to combat the false dichotomy set up by the media, "economy versus lives." This would finally become understood, I figured.

One other key point was always missing from the narrative emanating from the media. Without minimizing the dangers and the tragic death toll, there was in fact cause for optimism. At this point, far more was now known compared to the early months, especially that the overwhelming majority of Americans were not at serious risk. Kids were generally not in serious danger. Some people already had immune protection, and a large percentage of infections were so mild they were asymptomatic. And for the high-risk population, extraordinary progress was being made on vaccines.

Inexplicably, Dr. Fauci and others were not transmitting that positive data. That omission, in my mind, was an enormous, unforgivable failure of the public health leadership. Instead of showing the accumulated body of evidence that would calm people, and the decades of known biology, most public health officials decided to stress the unknown, adding to the public's panic. In my mind, one way to alleviate that fear was to have the president exhibit knowledge about the facts.

I then had another meeting with Jared. In his office, we discussed what seemed to be an emerging role on the president's team.

I needed to be very clear about my role—I was not going to be a mouthpiece for anyone. This was my primary concern. No one would tell me what to say, period, and anyone who really knew me understood that.

"First," I declared, "I want to make sure you know what you're getting with me. I will never say anything that isn't correct and true. I will never agree with someone else's comments if that isn't correct, no matter who tells me to. And I will never sign on to a group statement that I do not agree with."

"That's exactly why we want you here," he replied, without hesitation. "We know that."

I was impressed, thrilled really, because I saw he was sincere. And then Kushner said something else that caught me by surprise.

"If you become visible, if it becomes publicly known that you are here, they will try to destroy you. I am worried about that."

I never expected that from him, and for an instant it threw me. I was a health policy scholar, with an unassailable CV, right? Health policy analysis had been my job at Hoover for more than fifteen years. And I knew the data cold. How would reporters be able to destroy me? Still, I was taken aback.

"Thanks for that. How about this? For now, I would like to try to advise from my home back in California."

"Great, let's try that. Thank you for coming."

* * * * *

After only a few days, it became obvious the arrangement wouldn't work. The president and the White House were issuing statements and decisions were being made, and it was impossible to be meaningfully involved. I was communicating with Washington, but being out of sight along with the time difference minimized any real impact. The American people needed to hear from the president, and he in turn needed advice and input on how to provide his message against panic. I particularly needed to help him put forth the case against the lockdowns. Much of what was being said directly conflicted with the data, and it was confusing—and scaring—the public. Most importantly, people were dying.

Against all common sense, the Task Force's focus on stopping the spread of infections at all costs—instead of protecting those known to be at highest risk—was abjectly failing. Whatever happened to the more limited goal of "flattening the curve" and avoiding hospital overcrowding? And since when was it even rational to think it was within our power to stop every…single…case? And beyond that, no one was talking about the enormous damage being done to families and children by the lockdowns.

Yes, the president initially had gone along with the lockdowns proposed by Fauci and Birx, the "fifteen days to slow the spread," even though he had serious misgivings. But I still believe the reason that he kept repeating his one question—"Do you agree with the initial shutdown?"—whenever he asked questions about the pandemic was precisely because he still had misgivings about it. I always replied, "Yes, it was a reasonable strategy at the time. We had very little data, everyone thought the fatality rate was extremely high, and it was a temporary closure." Months before I arrived, by midspring, he understood the disastrous impact of the lockdowns, the destruction of families, businesses, and ordinary people's lives. As he pushed for vaccine development and opening schools and businesses, the conflict was obvious between his view and what Fauci and Birx told the states.

Meanwhile, the Task Force, particularly Dr. Fauci in his media appearances, kept focusing on what *might* happen, stressing what we didn't know with absolute certainty, rather than underscoring what we did know about the virus based on months of evidence, including the most fundamental biology. The Task Force was failing to communicate any clinical medical perspective, never clarifying that rare complications are just that—rare. Even worse, the media was sensationalizing every new piece of information. The panic itself had become another contagion.

I reluctantly decided to fly back to Washington. I packed a single suitcase, not knowing how long I would stay. I thought I would offer input but would remain behind the scenes. If I ended up becoming public, I tried to reassure myself, my credentials and emphasis on facts, not politics, would tamp down any controversy. All of the insanity I witnessed over the summer had prompted me to revisit a book I hadn't read for decades. At the last minute, I grabbed it—the only book I packed in my briefcase—for my flight to Washington. That book, *Alice's Adventures in Wonderland*, sat on my hotel nightstand, remaining unopened for the next four months, perhaps because it turned out I was living it every day and night anyway.

After arriving in Washington and checking back into the Willard Hotel, I walked to a nearby restaurant to grab dinner. On the way, I passed the gates to the White House grounds and peered through to the East Wing and North Lawn. It was surreal to think that I was here, part of that world.

My phone rang as I waited outside for my table.

"Hello. Is this Dr. Atlas?"

"Yes, this is Dr. Atlas."

"This is the White House operator. Are you available to speak with the president?"

"Yes, of course."

"Please hold."

About twenty seconds of silence passed. The operator's voice returned. "The president of the United States."

After a short wait, a familiar voice came on the line. President Trump warmly welcomed me back to Washington. We had a very friendly, fifteen-minute conversation. The president was gracious, thanking me more than once for leaving California and my family to come to the nation's capital.

"There is nothing more important to the country right now than addressing this crisis," I said. "Thank you, Mr. President, for asking me for input. I hope I can at least provide something beneficial to you and your team."

He casually mentioned several different topics during the call. Among those, he interspersed a series of questions about the pandemic. Again, he asked me about the initial lockdown, about testing, and about closing schools. He darted from topic to topic, from person to person, some directly related to the pandemic, and others not. At one point, he asked, "What about Fauci? Is it too late?" I replied, "Well, Mr. President, he's going to keep talking. He just recommended that everyone wear goggles."

Above all, the president stressed that even though the virus was extremely serious, continuing the lockdowns was shattering people, destroying the economy, keeping kids out of school, devastating small businesses.

The president then memorably said, "I'm sure you will teach me many things while you're here. But there is only one thing you'll learn from me. Only one. You will learn how vicious, how biased, how unfair the media is. You already know they are the fake news. But you have no idea how badly. That is the one thing that you will learn from me here."

The call ended, and I thought to myself, "Sure, I know the media is biased. I am fine with that. I know what I'm talking about, and I'm not here for political reasons. No problem."

I walked into the restaurant and ordered a glass of wine and a steak, totally naive and completely unprepared to be at the center of a national political maelstrom.

* * * * *

The night I returned to serve as special advisor, I called Rader to tell him I was in Washington. John gave me my first task—a session that same night with Derek Lyons. John told me, "You need to convince Derek. He has his doubts about the lockdowns, he is very analytical, and he is open to understanding the data underlying what you are saying. You need to be able to convince him."

Derek was the president's staff secretary. A brilliant, soft-spoken, Harvard-trained lawyer, a gentleman in the true sense of the term, Derek was the last word on documents drafted for presidential signature. Among other duties, he was also at the end of the long chain of people who edited the president's remarks for press briefings and other public events. Rader insisted that I go through the data on the pandemic, justifying my rationale that we should protect those at risk, with heightened urgency and increased diligence, while opening up the lockdowns for healthy, lower risk people.

I spent more than two hours explaining the key points about the pandemic to Derek, answering dozens of his challenging questions. From then on, I rarely missed a day of talking with Derek, usually because he was still testing me on some point I had made. More often than not, he was sitting behind his desk, looking at the raw data himself. I soon became a fixture in the Staff Sec office, often joking with his assistants that I would move my desk into their small, shared space adjacent to Derek's office. When I really became frustrated—a frequent occurrence—I would head into Derek's office, apologizing for occupying his valuable time with my complaints. Eventually, no apology was needed; it was such a regular event. And besides, he was just as frustrated, often tightly gripping a baseball bat in his hands as we shared our incredulity about the insanity unfolding before our eyes.

True, the president explicitly agreed with my views that lockdowns were extremely harmful to working families and children. And yes, the most influential among his inner circle already supported my policy recommendations—or at least repeatedly reassured me that they agreed. But during that very first week, it became clear my task would not be easy.

* * * * *

Kushner planned that I would join both the "COVID Huddle," generally held three times per week, and the Task Force meetings. But not yet. He was acutely aware that Dr. Birx would feel threatened. For the first few COVID Huddle gatherings, I was literally kept out of the room. Instead I was set up on a telephone outside to merely listen in. I was even advised to be discreet in displaying my newly assigned White House badge, out of caution that Dr. Birx might spot it and realize I wasn't going to be a temporary visitor. That seemed extreme. "They must really think she will go ballistic!" I thought to myself. I had never experienced this sort of concern. I hadn't heard of Dr. Birx before she appeared on the Task Force next to the president, but I checked for myself. A couple of points added significant insight into her mindset. She had a thirty-five-year career in government positions, as it turned out, and virtually all of it was focused on HIV/AIDS. Before that she served as director of CDC's Division of Global HIV/AIDS. In the military before that, she worked on "increasing the efficiency and effectiveness of the U.S. Military's HIV/AIDS efforts through inter- and intra-agency collaboration."

Given the remarkable sensitivity to her reaction, I also asked how she had been appointed—that seemed to be a bit of a mystery to everyone. I was told by Jared, more than once, "Dr. Birx is 100 percent MAGA!"—as if that should make all the other issues somehow less important. Secretary Azar denied appointing her during his stint running the Task Force. I was told by the VP's chief of staff, Marc Short, that Pence "inherited her" when he took over as chair of the Task Force. No one seemed to know.

One more thing caught my eye. Birx had worked in Fauci's lab and then been the research assistant of Redfield in the late 1980s. Once she was in a position of authority over research funding in her role in Obama's "President's Emergency Plan for AIDS Relief," or

PEPFAR, Redfield received millions of dollars for his lab. This was not exactly a well-rounded team of independent, diverse voices for designing health policy for this pandemic.

The situation with keeping me hidden was bizarre, but I put it down to my unfamiliarity with people in politics. I already knew I had nothing in common with those who had held government jobs with multiple layers of staff under them for decades. I also failed to realize how much that difference mattered.

Even though it was strange to hide my badge, I was glad enough to do so. From the moment I arrived in the West Wing, I too wanted to avoid causing a stir. In fact, that's exactly why I initially told Kushner I did not want to be part of the Task Force. What would be the point? I already knew what most on the Task Force thought—shut down everything, close schools, isolate everyone, in an attempt to stop the cases, no matter the harms. Correction: The whole country already knew what the Task Force thought. Then again, that's why I was brought in, because I disagreed with that narrow view, specifically because I understood the lockdowns were destructive.

The views of Drs. Fauci and Birx, and the rest of their group, had already been on display for more than six months. I felt it was extremely naive to think that these people were open to changing their minds on fundamental positions. They were fixated on lockdowns, school closures, and stopping COVID cases, no matter the economic and human costs. I had already been quite visible in disagreeing publicly with what I considered to be their grossly misguided policies. After all, they had no problem contradicting the desire of the president of the United States to end the lockdowns. Why in the world would they be convinced by me, a total outsider?

After an initial—and quick—meeting with Dr. Birx, I saw that Kushner's concerns were fully warranted. She seemed threatened right away by my presence. She was noticeably uneasy, even though I told her, "I'm just here to help in any way I can." She instantly asked, with slight hesitancy in her voice, "How long will you be there?" I said it wasn't clear, which was certainly true. My White House badge, a sign of some permanence, was tucked inside my laptop case.

Dr. Birx then warned, "There are many people around here who think the pandemic is not even serious. I just want you to know that." I was taken aback by her comment—I thought it was odd. So many deaths, the world was literally paralyzed, and people in the White House didn't take it seriously? "Well, it's true that she's already been here for six months," I thought. Still, I had my doubts that she was right. I had certainly not perceived that in any of my discussions so far. I swiftly dismissed her notion that I myself might be one of those individuals. I stressed that I knew it was very serious, of course; the biggest health care crisis in a century. That was not even a question. I explicitly stated that the issue was "how to manage it best, to save lives." Dr. Birx nodded affirmatively.

That first chat with Dr. Birx was soon followed by a longer meeting that Kushner had asked me to set up. I showed up a few minutes early and waited in her office. She entered wearing her mask, very atypical of most others walking around in the West Wing.

I stood to say "hello" and asked, "Would you like me to put on a mask?" "No, no," she said waving her hand. "I have been traveling in areas where there is high activity; that's why I have my mask on." She removed it. That naturally led to a discussion on masks.

"Just curious," I asked, "what study is the most important one to show masks are effective?"

"The hair salon study!" she replied confidently.

I knew the study well, having already dissected it in detail with a few epidemiologists before I set foot in Washington. My colleagues had all laughed at it. It was poorly done, and the conclusions were not valid. It was an embarrassment that it had been published prominently on the CDC website, let alone cited in the media by experts.

There was tension in the room as I mentioned, in as diplomatic a way as I could muster, some concerns about the study's design. This was what would be charitably described as a clinical report, but not solid science. Two hair stylists were working in a salon. One became ill with COVID, and she subsequently infected the other while still working for several days. The clients wore masks when they were in the salon. Many were later simply asked over the phone if they contracted the infection. "Of course, the clients were always facing directly away from the hair stylist," which was even acknowledged in the paper, reducing exposure. More importantly, I pointed out that most were not even in the shop very long.

Dr. Birx smiled and said, "Well, Scott, you may not realize it but women sit there for several hours getting their hair done."

"Yes, I do realize that," I said, politely adding, "I hope it's OK that I question it. I am a pretty direct person. I hope you don't mind if I disagree."

"I have no problem with you disagreeing." And she added what was to become her common refrain, "I am all about the data!"

We spoke for a bit longer, and then I left. Right away, I looked up the study on the CDC website to be sure I had remembered it correctly. Indeed, half the subjects were in the salon for only fifteen minutes, total. No one was in the shop more than forty-five minutes—not "hours" as Dr. Birx assumed. Not only did they all minimize exposure by facing away from the stylist as their hair was being cut, half of the participants barely met CDC criteria for the minimum amount of time that defined "exposure."

There were other important questions. No other stylists working with the two infected hair stylists, Stylist A and Stylist B, all mingling without masks, developed COVID symptoms. Did they catch the infection? None were tested, so we don't know. Close at-home contacts of Stylist A became infected, but the two close at-home contacts of Stylist B did not develop COVID. Perhaps that implies that Stylist B was simply not a spreader of the infection, regardless of mask wearing. These were obvious questions that should make one hesitate, if one looks at it critically, as a scientist should.

Dr. Birx did not seem to know about several additional methodological problems. More than half of the clients were never even tested for the virus. Without proof by testing, we have no idea if there was a difference between the number of clients who became infected and those who did not. More than 25 percent were not even contacted for a phone interview to see if they had COVID.

I didn't feel good that I had been correct. I had already known that the study she cited was nowhere near to being definitive as Dr. Birx had claimed. I was further alarmed that Dr. Birx had dug in on her belief when challenged, and showed no awareness at the meeting about some important flaws in the study she most relied on. Yet this was the study she herself had cited as the most significant evidence proving that masks were effective. Another anxiety-provoking moment—in the "this is really bad" sense—had come to pass. It was still my first week on the job.

*   *   *   *   *

I needed to figure out exactly how to proceed strategically. I had met Dr. Birx, but that wasn't very promising. I had been told to hide my badge and listen in on COVID Huddle meetings from Kushner's office. On my arrival, I was handed an earlier draft of an overall strategy speech for President Trump to deliver and asked to totally revise it ASAP. I included an update on what we had learned about the virus, then outlined the fundamentals of a strategy centered on three points: increased protection of the high-risk population; carefully monitoring hospitals and ICUs in all states; and guiding businesses, transportation, and schools to safely reopen. The speech included many specifics, but it was never delivered.

Meanwhile, I was also still looking at the data myself—as much as I could, every morning beginning at 6:00, whenever I had a chance throughout the day, and every night after dinner, until at least 1:00 a.m. Concurrently, I was going back and forth with epidemiologists from the West Coast, the East Coast, and Europe on a daily basis, dissecting every meaningful research paper that had come out in the previous forty-eight hours.

But that was just scratching the surface. For several months, there had been a period when the COVID press briefings were significantly reduced. A number of conflicts had been generated in previous briefings, including misstatements about treatments and other snags that had been detrimental to the discussion and fed into the frenzy of misinformation and doubt. The faces of the Task Force, Drs. Birx and Fauci, had stood by silently during the president's conjectures about drinking disinfectant and the efficacy of various drugs in a way that was confusing and contributed to public fear. At least, that was my recollection.

My recommendation to the White House, even before I arrived in Washington, was very different. Instead of remaining less visible, the president himself needed to stand up and personally discuss the data in detail. That way, Americans would see that the administration was taking things seriously and that the president himself was fully briefed and closely monitoring the latest developments.

To help accomplish that, I was asked on a daily basis about the newest trends around the country and what was important to emphasize. It was not a simple task, since the dataset was almost unlimited and changing every day. I did not just accept the simplistic compilations that Dr. Birx received and partly distributed. Many times, I wanted to illustrate more relevant and specific comparisons or drill down on data that had not been compiled accurately by governments. I frequently discussed specific points with the scientists actually doing the research.

I also sometimes requested original source data from people with whom I had developed relationships. These were concerned citizens from all over the country—accomplished, mathematically oriented Americans and researchers who, like me, now devoted their days to pandemic analysis. They remained "on call" when I had specific questions or when I wanted something directly compared, day or night. That became especially valuable, since some of the data being distributed by Dr. Birx on cases, hospitalizations, and deaths per day seemed to be drawn from layman-level websites like "worldometer," a compiler that may or may not have included accurate numbers on its website, and opaque state-government sources. Most data on those websites did not accurately reflect peaks and trends due to misregistration of episode dates because of later batch recording, or inadequate depth of analysis—problems widely known outside the White House, but apparently known to no one inside, including the Task Force.

I also made sure that Kayleigh McEnany, the White House press secretary, understood the data. I often went to her office with stacks of scientific publications, explaining the data so she was fully updated and accurate in her words to the astonishingly hostile press corps. In this new model of briefings, the president himself was detailing facts. Even though many people contributed to the president's remarks, my input was requested 24/7, real-time. I did my best to ensure that no mistake was made on anything I added. Every source was defined; absolutely no uncertainty was acceptable, or it was discarded.

The main reason for my presence was to impact policy, not just try to help the president and the country accurately understand the current status of the pandemic. After all, I was a health policy expert, not an epidemiologist or virologist. My expertise, my role, was to devise a set of policies that minimized the harms of the pandemic—including the harms of the policies themselves. Americans would have been frightened if they had realized that there was no one on the Task Force with any medical background who understood, or was even concerned with, these impacts. To delegate policy to people solely concerned with stopping the infection, without any understanding of the destruction of the lockdowns, would have been reckless.

But that's exactly what happened. In enacting lockdowns without evaluating the secondary health effects of those harsh policies, the fundamental principles of public health were violated They failed to consider the total health impact of the policies and the pandemic; they also failed to protect those most vulnerable to those harms—children, the poor, and the elderly. That inappropriate commandeering of policy by a narrow focus on stopping the spread of the infection and nothing else is the main reason so many people died during this pandemic, why so many families were destroyed, and why so many disastrous public health consequences will be endured by young and old for decades.

The president believed that the country should reopen. Months earlier, in March 2020, he had warned, "The cure cannot be worse than the disease." He opposed lockdowns and understood at a gut level their disastrous harms. The White House had already gone so far as to produce documents emphasizing reopening. In April 2020, their reopening guide stated, "A long-term nationwide shutdown is not sustainable and would inflict wide-ranging harm on the health and wellbeing of our citizens."

Yet that fundamental policy of the president's was ignored, overtly contradicted almost daily by Dr. Birx, who represented the White House Task Force to governors and regional media while visiting states. At times, she was accompanied by Vice President Pence, thereby providing an implicit endorsement. Fauci meanwhile was all over the map in his statements.

By the time I arrived, lockdowns had already been implemented throughout the country for months—including strict business restrictions and school closures as well as quarantines of healthy, asymptomatic people. Those lockdowns were continually pushed, successfully, by Drs. Fauci and Birx to nearly all governors and throughout the media. Those policies—the Birx-Fauci lockdowns—were widely implemented, and they were destroying America's children and families. Meanwhile, hundreds of thousands of deaths kept piling up, including tens of thousands of elderly Americans—*their policies were in place and were failing*. Yet, that failure was not only disregarded, it was taken to mean that the lockdowns were needed even more.

One confusion that was amplified by the media was the division of responsibility for the management of the pandemic. Being a federalist system, the pandemic response was a joint effort between the federal government, the states, and local municipalities. In a practical sense, the federal government provided support for the state-based decisions, which were then implemented on a local level. All on-the-ground policies were the purview of the governors, the chief executive of each state, not the president. That authority was not "delegated" by President Trump—it is the constitutional

SCOTT W. ATLAS, MD

authority of the governor in our federalist system, and it was appropriately demanded by each governor. But of course, with that
authority necessarily comes responsibility. Each state designed its
own lockdowns, mandates, school closures, and personal restrictions, and each governor bears responsibility for the outcomes of
those policies.

That does not mean the president had no national leadership
role—he clearly did. The vice president's Task Force also had a significant leadership role, beyond its concern with logistics regarding
the production and delivery of supplies. The Task Force provided
strategic advice to the governors and state public health officials.
The problem was that the president's message—end the lockdowns
and use a focused protection of the high-risk—was directly contrary
to the lockdown message of the Task Force. Allowing the national
policy message to be contrary to the message of the president of
the United States was a gross error. It allowed the destructive lockdown policy to remain in place and presented a picture of a chaotic
national leadership in the pandemic response. Those who advised
the president to allow that to continue did him and the nation a
tremendous disservice.

CHAPTER 4.
The Mad Hatter's Tea Party

After getting the feel of the West Wing environment, I entered the Task Force meetings in mid-August, at the direction of Jared. It was against my better judgment, and I told him so. Their single-minded advice for stopping COVID-19 was firmly established; that was clear. In my mind, it was fantasy to think that these entrenched bureaucrats would be amenable to convincing by me, a total outsider. And they obviously did not acknowledge or care about the consequences of prolonged lockdowns. I dreaded the idea of what would inevitably be frustration and conflict, with virtually no chance of positive outcome. But I said OK. I wanted to be cooperative, and I also knew the VP was very welcoming to my presence.

My first revelation about the Task Force was that the public perception was far off base, both in terms of its structure and how it functioned. The Task Force was run entirely by Vice President Pence. The president was not part of the Task Force; in fact, he never once attended those meetings during my time in the White House. I always laughed at press reports trying to portray that as a sudden change, an alarming new development. The president never spoke with the Task Force as a group, to my knowledge, during my four months in Washington. To underscore that clear separation, I always sensed relief, along with some annoyance, in Kushner's voice when he would answer, "That's the domain of the vice president," whenever I relayed concerns from angry governors about policies emanating from Dr. Birx.

In turn, unless a Task Force member had a separate meeting with the president or was part of the president's press briefings, the member had no direct interaction with him. That also meant you were not visible to the public in that capacity. That lack of visibility was clearly a sore spot for some who had previously been highly visible at his side in public view. Both Dr. Fauci and Dr. Birx described feeling "marginalized" once I arrived. In truth, though, well before I arrived at the end of July, the president had already stopped speaking with Birx or Fauci. In emails coming to light now, Birx wrote, "Tony and I did not brief the President nor speak to the President between 22 April and the end of July beyond one vaccine briefing in July." Birx later went further on the Sunday talk shows, expressing personal dismay—shock!—that "information she had not provided made its way to the President," as if she ought to be the sole purveyor of crucial information to the president.

In practice, the operations of the Task Force had separate components: 1) medical-related assessments and advice; and 2) concrete deliverables, both production and logistics, involving safety equipment, testing, emergency medical resources, drugs, and vaccines. A separate set of people provided updates on the economy, including the state of operations in businesses and schools.

The part of the Task Force dealing with deliverables and operations functioned impressively well, at least during the time I was there. Groups reported in detail on protective equipment, testing, hospital personnel, bed capacity increases, and other related equipment needed to handle the pandemic, much of which derived from invoking the emergency Defense Production Act. Logistics underlying the distribution of these elements seemed highly organized under the direction of Federal Emergency Management Agency Administrator Pete Gaynor and Admiral John Polowczyk. Specific, mostly sensible agency directives were also generated; for instance, Seema Verma, head of the Centers for Medicare and Medicaid Services (CMS), worked thoughtfully on policies to improve nursing home operations. Others continually updated the group on important progress with Operation Warp Speed (OWS), the vaccine development program under HHS Secretary Alex Azar, especially its private sector partnerships to expedite drug and vaccine development, led by Dr. Moncef Slaoui.

The medical side of the Task Force was an entirely different story. On that side, Dr. Birx was in charge. In her role as Task Force coordinator, she summarized the state of the pandemic for the vice president. She was nearly the entire public representation of the Task Force outside Washington, because she was the one who flew around the country, at times with the VP, meeting with local authorities and appearing on regional media. On these visits, Birx directly advised the governors and public health officials. Each state also regularly received her summary of trends including specific advice on personal behavior, mandates, and restrictions on businesses and schools. Those updates were sometimes also distributed to the Task Force and COVID Huddles, especially if any upcoming event would be occurring in those states.

That advice was under the domain of Dr. Birx herself, as Task Force Coordinator; I had zero input. The fact is, her policy advice was just that—advice. It was to be implemented at the sole discretion of the states and local municipalities—and indeed it was. Governors used the advice of Dr. Birx and especially the CDC guidelines to justify their chosen policies, no doubt. Contrary to the way it was portrayed in the media, very little on-the-ground policy was truly under the control of the federal government, aside from international travel and other specialized areas under the jurisdiction of federal authority.

Task Force meetings were held in the Situation Room. However, that name does not designate just one room—it refers to a set of conference rooms on the ground floor of the West Wing equipped with secure telecommunication capabilities. Every Task Force meeting was held in the same specific room inside the complex, with an overflow room nearby, along with videoconferencing connections to dozens more in other government agencies and locations.

Each Task Force meeting began with spotting the handout packets at everyone's place around the oval conference table, including the set agenda. Approximately eight to ten of us had assigned seats at the table, seating chart distributed in advance. A dozen or so others stood around the periphery of the room, and a nearby overflow room was also filled. Even more were connected digitally to the meeting from various agencies. We would casually exchange pleasantries for a few minutes while waiting, and then Vice President Pence would enter. All stood formally as he entered with his staff. He then thanked everyone for attending and asked that everyone be seated. The VP was always beaming with positivity, a model of running such gatherings, I thought, as he focused on encouraging participation while efficiently going through the agenda.

The mode of the VP was to hold the meetings in a very orderly fashion. He opened every meeting with very gracious thanks to the group, including all those connected digitally, and heartfelt appreciation to each person as they finished presenting their agenda item. Every item was held open for all who wanted to comment. Likewise, every meeting ended with his profuse gratitude for their efforts and accomplishments, a very sincerely delivered "thank you so much all for your extremely hard work on behalf of the American people and the president."

As I later witnessed, several meetings also ended with explicit appreciation from the VP to those around the table for maintaining a positive outlook with the media. Perhaps because I was still unaccustomed to the insincere statements of politicians, this was shocking to me, as this praise often occurred even after I had watched multiple TV interviews by these same people being overtly critical of the president's policies and undermining public trust by blatantly contradicting the administration's statements about progress and time lines on crucial deliverables like vaccines. Many times I found myself looking around the room, wondering if I was the only one who had just heard what was said and was aware of the reality.

Medical and science issues were principally discussed by five people, including myself, who regularly sat at the table. In that room, the vice president often referred to us informally as Deb, Tony, Bob, Brett, and Scott. Each of us had different roles, and there seemed to be a relatively fixed seating position at the table. Dr. Birx (Deb) was the titular Task Force coordinator and was always positioned to the right of VP Pence, who sat at the head of the table. To her right was Dr. Fauci (Tony); Dr. Robert Redfield (Bob), the director of the CDC; Admiral Giroir (Brett), also a medical doctor and the testing czar; and me, the special advisor to the president.

The rest of the seating varied, because other members were not present at every meeting, depending on their personal schedules and the agenda. Seema Verma, head of CMS, was regularly present. Surgeon-General Jerome Adams, Secretary Azar, and other agency directors or cabinet members were only occasionally there. I think I saw the head of the FDA, Dr. Stephen Hahn, at only one Task Force meeting. Around the room, high-level staff, members of related agencies and departments, and some members of the administration's political team were regular or occasional attendees. Several of those in the West Wing whom I considered rational actors had given up on attending out of frustration and fatigue with the inane statements bandied about. Needless to say, there were plenty of potential leakers to the press.

After the initial welcome from the VP, Dr. Birx was always asked to start. She gave her spiel after first smiling broadly and accepting with a loud, "Thank you, Mr. Vice President," going proudly through her tables of numbers and charts, many of which had no actionable significance. That was her primary role in that room; she was the presenter of the week's COVID trends to the group, color-coded to fit preconceived, arbitrary categories. When I say arbitrary, I mean that Birx assigned specific ranges to different categories, even though there was no proven importance to those specific numbers. For instance, states were divided into colors, based on their percentage of positive tests from the testing each state had conducted. In August, she was dividing states into three colors: "green" for less than 5 percent positive tests, "red" for states with greater than 10 percent test positivity, and "yellow" for those 5-to-10 percent positive. Her system became more "detailed" later. "Dark green" states by definition had less than 3 percent positive tests; "light green" corresponded to between 3 and 5 percent positive; "yellow states" had a 5-to-8 percent test positivity; "orange" indicated states with 8-to-10 percent, and "red states" meant greater than 10 percent. More categories must have meant more scientific to her, I guessed.

It wasn't just that those categories had no known predictive significance. They also assumed, erroneously, that each state used the same standardized criteria for determining who was tested. Even if that color coding was used by others, it had no clear scientific meaning or significance. To me, it reflected the way a naive person who simply wanted to categorize for the sake of categorizing might think. Watching Birx attach such solemn significance to these arbitrarily chosen, non-standardized categories, and then pretending that more detailed significance came from dividing into more refined yet still arbitrary categories, brought to mind flashes of scenes from Joseph Heller's *Catch-22*. Birx also updated everyone on her travels around the country, providing anecdotal assessments as to whether people were obeying mitigation measures, or if public health officials had issues with testing; if necessary, she would call in from the road. The rest of the agenda changed every week.

Fauci's role surprised me the most. Most of the country, indeed the entire world, assumed that Fauci occupied a directorial role in the Trump administration's Task Force. I had also thought that from viewing the news. That perception initially made sense, stemming from the visible presence of Fauci at the president's briefings early on in the pandemic, back in the late winter and spring of 2020. But those appearances at the podium had long been discontinued. The misunderstanding of Dr. Fauci's role derived mainly from his nearly ubiquitous presence and solo interviews on national and international media. To my knowledge, no one in the White House filtered his interview requests. Any implication that he was somehow held back from appearing in the media provoked laughter in the West Wing. It was a running joke in the White House; most people marveled that he could even find the time to conduct so many interviews.

The public presumption of Dr. Fauci's leadership role on the Task Force itself, though, could not have been more incorrect. Fauci held massive sway with the public, but he was not in charge of anything specific on the Task Force. He served mainly as a channel for updates on the trials of vaccines and drugs. That is not to say Fauci directed the vaccine development; he did not. The vaccine development was directed by the highly capable Dr. Slaoui, hand in hand with the partner companies. The vaccine and other logistics were under the proficient leadership of General Gus Perna, Lt. General Paul Ostrowski, and others, including agencies like FEMA; the drug clinical trials and the team from industry were under the direction of Francis Collins; the entirety of Operation Warp Speed remained under the umbrella of responsibilities of Secretary Azar and his team, including the highly capable Paul Mango.

Fauci passed on information to the Task Force about the status of clinical trial enrollment, for instance how many people in which demographic had been enrolled into the vaccine or drug trials. But like everyone else, he had no advance knowledge about the results of vaccine trials, because those were in a "black box" until the outside board of experts made their intermittent safety and efficacy assessments. Likewise, drug treatment results were compiled and released by the researchers and drug companies themselves, in concert with the FDA. A bigger surprise was that Fauci did not present scientific research on the pandemic to the group that I witnessed. Likewise, I never heard him speak about his own critical analysis of any published research studies. This was stunning to me. Aside from intermittent status updates about clinical trial enrollments, Fauci served the Task Force by offering an occasional comment or update on vaccine trial participant totals, mostly when the VP would turn to him and ask.

Evident from my first encounter was what appeared to be a functioning troika of "medical experts" composed of Drs. Birx, Fauci, and Redfield. They shared thought processes and views to an uncanny level. One depressing commonality was that none of them showed detailed knowledge of ongoing scientific literature on the pandemic. As opposed to what I had experienced with my colleagues in academic research centers, I never witnessed any of them provide any detailed critique of any journal publication. Unlike scientists with whom I had worked for decades, I never saw them voice any critical assessment, methodological or otherwise, of the pitfalls of any published studies. That analytical process is an extremely important part of evaluating medical research. Likewise, none of the three ever brought scientific publications into the meetings that I attended. And unlike other doctors I had worked with, none showed familiarity with clinical medicine or had any clinical perspective on medical journal publications or any facility with clinical terminology in meetings I attended during my time in Washington.

All this was surprising to me, because that was exactly what I perceived to be the role of those with medical science backgrounds. For example, in advance of every meeting, I went through all relevant medical publications, having discussed them when necessary with outside colleagues to make sure I understood any flaws or pitfalls that might have led to wrong or invalid conclusions. That is how a scientist approaches a scientific question. I also made sure to bring dozens of relevant papers to every meeting, stacks of them, that would shed light on the topics to be discussed.

I also noticed that there was virtually no disagreement among them. It was an amazing consistency, as though there were an agreed-upon complicity—even though some of their statements were so patently simplistic or erroneous that others in the room, even those without medical backgrounds, sometimes felt compelled to make corrections. I found myself grateful to people like Seema Verma; Marc Short, the VP's chief of staff; and others who occasionally spoke up to challenge their conclusions—grateful, because at some meetings, I felt burned out, simply unable to muster the energy to yet again correct something so unmistakably wrong. That happened most commonly when selective correlations were assumed to be cause and effect, like a non-scientist might conclude (for example, pointing to the correlation of cases with the timing of a mandate in one state but ignoring that comparison in a different state where it did not correlate).

Even on those strikingly unsound conclusions, Drs. Birx, Fauci, and Redfield virtually always agreed, literally never challenging one other.

Dr. Giroir at times raised questions, but his willingness to buck the others was very limited. My sense was that Giroir, more than anything, wanted to fit into the "team," hence he usually agreed with the others, although he privately worked well with me. Giroir rigidly adhered to all rules. He stood literally at attention when Pence walked into the Situation Room, understandable given that Giroir was always in uniform. Once, I forgot to remove my phone from my pocket when I entered, and Giroir was outraged, frantically ordering me to remove it from the area ASAP. But of all of us in the group, only one ever raised her voice and interrupted repeatedly, behavior that eventually prompted me to calmly request on more than one occasion, "Excuse me, can I please finish?" That person was Dr. Birx.

CHAPTER 5
The Politics of Testing

By the time I arrived at the end of July, the administration had already developed a massive testing capacity from scratch. Nearly a million tests per day were being conducted. The effort was led by Admiral Giroir, who was assigned the thankless task of overseeing that project.

I understood why the VP was so excited when he had displayed that simplistic chart on my first visit. And over the next weeks the administration continued to successfully facilitate and distribute tens of millions of point-of-care PCR tests and, later, rapid antigen tests. This was a significant accomplishment, but it was clear from the beginning that the White House did not understand how or when to use testing. To my thinking, it was a response to political pressure more than anything else.

From my very first meeting in the Oval Office back in July and again over subsequent meetings, President Trump expressed great frustration about testing. It was easy to see why. You could not turn on the news, even the most superficial talk show, without the lead story admonishing the administration for "the lack of testing." For months, the country had been inundated with that message—not just from public health types who had now become household names, but from every pundit, talk show host, and news anchor. It became pure groupthink. Celebrities who had no understanding or expertise at all were now stridently opining about the unquestionable urgency of massive, widespread, on-demand testing.

Reminiscent of stock market frenzies, esoteric technical terms that had formerly been unknown to the public like "contact tracing" now became common parlance. Testing for this virus had turned into a national, indeed, international obsession. And to me, that obsession was not just misguided, it was harmful, creating more fear, more frenzy, more irrational policies. Yes, testing was an essential tool in the pandemic. And yes, months before I was involved in any way in Washington, there had been a failure to develop and deliver enough tests when they were needed the most. But by the time I came to DC at the end of July, a massive capacity to test had been quickly developed. The problem now was that it was not being leveraged to save lives. Schools and businesses were closed; people were cowering in their homes. Meanwhile, older people kept dying by the thousands.

Criticizing the administration about testing was more than a natural extension of that obsessive mindset. It was low-hanging fruit for the president's political opponents. There had been almost no preexisting testing capacity from the outset, so naturally it would take some time to meet the challenge. The obsessive demand for testing rapidly escalated into a hyperpartisan issue. I remembered Pelosi's mantra—"test, test, test; trace, trace, trace!"—as if she, or any politician for that matter, had any understanding of the appropriate testing policy. She was not alone, though. That mantra was echoed on every news network, regardless of political leaning. No dissenting opinion was even visible to most Americans.

That political heat provoked the expected reaction in the White House. Long before my arrival, testing became Priority Number One. Beyond an important public health policy question, it was an election season, and a contentious one at that. This environment elevated testing into *the* priority of the president's closest counselors, his political advisors at the highest levels, and operationally, therefore, the vice president's Task Force. Presumably, like all politicians, the president was politically motivated, too.

The conflict, the misjudgment about issues like testing and other advice coming out of the Task Force, occurred when the president was swayed too much by his political advisors instead of believing in his own common sense. That advice matched the message of the Task Force, especially that coming from Redfield and Birx, whose decision-making background was tied almost exclusively to testing. That was one of the many problems stemming from the HIV backgrounds of Birx and Redfield. SARS2 had already spread to millions, and it spread by breathing in close proximity; the role and practical application of testing in a virus like HIV couldn't have been more different. In the end, it was easy to see how the advice to the president was to focus on testing.

Understandable for everyone, that is, except the president. He never agreed, because to him it made no sense. He couldn't understand why we would test people who were not sick. It was as simple as that. President Trump talked to me privately in the Oval Office about many different things, but almost always, our discussions came back to the subject of testing. The president spoke very bluntly and resorted to common sense rather than any data. He knew nothing specific about the medical rationale for testing. He went with his gut feeling and placed no filter on stating his opinions.

"Why are we testing healthy, younger people? Why don't we just test sick people?" he would ask.

"And if we test more, we find more cases. But those people aren't sick!" he would point out, exasperated, echoing what he said many times to the press.

And that seemed rather straightforward, on its face. His point was simple logic—test and you shall discover "cases," especially with COVID, since a large number, maybe half or more, of infections were asymptomatic. He was also correct that in clinical medicine, the definition of a "case"—a patient—is not generally based on a test seeking out something in a healthy, asymptomatic person. That is not how medicine is practiced, a point I tried to explain time and again to the Task Force troika of doctors. I had that perspective, because I am a doctor who has been an expert for decades on the significance of diagnostic tests showing abnormalities without symptoms. And wasn't it also important to consider that the overwhelming majority of people did not have a serious illness, even when symptomatic? As for mildly ill patients with COVID, "standard of care" for them was strict isolation, *with or without testing*.

Testing, though, was the way—the only way—to find infected people who had *no* symptoms. In high-risk settings, contagious people with asymptomatic infections would be critical to find, no doubt. But the goal, the rationale for testing, became a key point of confusion and disagreement. We needed to protect high-risk people, absolutely. The question was how. We knew who was at risk, so there were two alternatives: 1) *indirectly* protecting the "vulnerable" by confining and locking down everyone else, or 2) doing everything to protect high-risk people *directly*.

By the time I set foot in the White House, the nation, with few exceptions, had already been using the Birx-Fauci lockdown restrictions—the indirect strategy—for months. Why was there no admission that the lockdown strategy did not work? It undeniably failed to protect the elderly. Nursing home deaths were piling up, comprising up to 80 percent of total deaths in some states—and in the meantime the lockdown policy was destroying everyone and everything else. Einstein may or may not have said it, but everyone knew it: "The definition of insanity is doing the same thing over and over and expecting different results." Yet the strategy was to continue doubling down on the failed lockdowns that were devastating to so many, especially those outside the "elite." Reality was being denied, and that remains the case today. Regardless, the answer to the failure, the available tool for those all-in on stopping all cases, was more testing!

Unbeknownst to the White House, several top epidemiologists and infectious disease experts had opined that massive testing of healthy people in settings that were not high-risk was not appropriate at this stage of a pandemic. That was apparent to me from months of lengthy discussions with leading epidemiologists at Stanford and elsewhere. There were already tens of millions of Americans who had been infected; even the CDC estimated a tenfold larger number compared to the confirmed number, as verified by early studies on SARS2 antibodies. Contact tracing was also "futile" at this point, as Dr. Bhattacharya later wrote in a paper I distributed at a Task Force meeting. Contact tracing was a tool for newly emerging pandemics, new outbreaks perhaps. Oxford's Sunetra Gupta, a world-renowned epidemiologist, repeatedly stressed the lack of logic in mass testing at this stage and the irrationality of focusing on cases by positive tests. Moreover, PCR tests were detecting virus fragments or dead virus in people who were not even contagious. Yet no one in the Task Force would even entertain this discussion.

The question about the role of testing was fundamental. It wasn't simply surveillance for the purpose of knowledge—testing was the key to a strategic policy. It was not enough to consider testing through the limited prism of an epidemiologist, the way Birx and Fauci did (even though they, like me, are not epidemiologists). In medical practice, if you referred a patient with low back pain to a neurosurgeon, the most likely outcome was surgery. That's exactly why I always referred patients to neurologists first—they had more perspective. Some might think of the adage "to someone with a hammer, everything looks like a nail." Testing was the main tool in the epidemiology toolbox, their only tool, really. That was very limiting in defining its role in overall policymaking.

At this juncture, the testing was not being done to yield statistically valid surveillance information—a legitimate use of testing in the midst of a pandemic. This was diagnostic testing, with broad-reaching policy aims. In this pandemic, a positive test was a major driver of the policy of quarantining and isolating healthy people with low-risk profiles—shuttering businesses, closing schools— in short, a key to locking down the country. That's why health policy experts like myself with a broader scope of expertise than that of epidemiologists and basic scientists are needed. Because no one with a medical science background who also considered the impacts of the policies was advising the White House. That lack of perspective was the main source of the tunnel-vision focus on preventing the spread of infections to the exclusion of all other considerations.

It was baffling to me, an incomprehensible error of whoever assembled the Task Force, that there were zero public health policy experts and no experts with medical knowledge who also analyzed economic, social, and other broad public health impacts other than the infection itself. Shockingly, the broad public health perspective was never part of the discussion among the Task Force health advisors other than when I brought it up. Even more bizarre was that no one seemed to notice.

The president clearly understood that testing healthy people for a disease that did not make them sick made little sense and would only lead to confining them. I agreed with that common sense view, although with important exceptions, and sitting in the Oval Office I explained the absurd extension of the logic of "test, test, test." What was the "necessary" number, anyway? One million per day? Not even close. One hundred million per day? Nope. How about everyone in the country—330 million per day, every day. Even if you could accomplish that goal, the tests themselves were only a snapshot in time. Seconds later, any given person could become infected. So 330 million per day, every fifteen minutes—maybe that would satisfy the testing mania! No matter how many tests were performed, there would never be enough.

The need for increased testing, but in a smarter, more targeted way, still needed to be explained to the president. And I did just that, repeatedly, whenever I had a chance—in concise, short doses. As always, he listened intently. But he had no time or patience for a detailed presentation. That is one reason why we got along well. I was capable of speaking succinctly, articulating the bottom line. More importantly, he knew I spoke directly, no BS.

From day one, I always reminded myself—if, and whenever, the president of the United States asks for my opinion, I am going to give it.

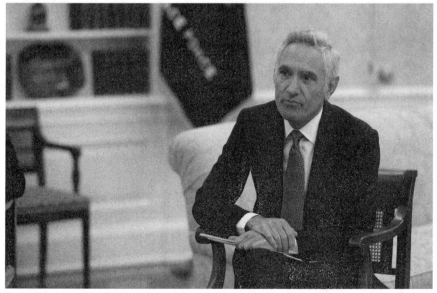

As usual, I sat in a chair directly in front of the president and listened closely to his pointed questions, so I could provide my best information and opinion. (*Credit: Official White House photographers*)

No holds barred—otherwise, what was I there for? Even on my very first visit to the Oval Office, when he complained about widespread testing, I bluntly told him, "You are a hamster on a wheel," knowing that others in the room would probably recoil at hearing that. But President Trump knew it, even repeating the phrase later himself.

There was, I explained, a more nuanced approach to the policy of testing. There were serious reasons to test, important reasons to actually *increase* testing, but in a strategic way. The question was how to leverage that testing capability to have the most impact—to save the most lives and to facilitate reopening the country, which was the right goal from both a health perspective and the president's stated policy. I thought my approach was obvious. This was simple logic, and it reiterated exactly what I had written months before: let's focus testing on where it really mattered, and *increase* it. High-risk environments, where high-risk people lived and worked. Nursing homes, a tinderbox of risk for its elderly, frail residents, were an obvious target. Knowing that cases were brought in by the staff, they needed to be tested, and tested far more frequently, perhaps every day. I also pushed for more point-of-care tests in places independent-living seniors frequented, like senior centers; visiting nurses taking care of seniors at home; and historically Black colleges and universities (HBCUs), where high-risk faculty members were more concentrated.

While the president understood and fully supported this, he remained frustrated, as did I, because his most trusted advisors didn't fully sign on to a strategic approach to testing. At one point he offhandedly remarked, "You'll have to convince my son-in-law of that." Naturally, Kushner and everyone else had been deferring to Fauci and Birx on all things medical. To make matters worse, the Fauci-Birx testing strategy was not merely unfocused; their strategy bizarrely prioritized more testing in the lowest-risk people and the lowest-risk environments—students and schools—while letting the deaths continue in nursing homes and assisted living facilities, where a once-per-week schedule was assumed to be effective.

Politics seemed to be the main driver of those in the inner circle advising the president—that was their job. But the politics were irrelevant to me. The frenzy about testing everyone, everywhere, at all times, including low-risk people in low-risk settings, was incorrect, illogical, and harmful.

The funny thing was that while almost everyone assumed the president was only making excuses, somehow covering up for an "inadequate" testing capacity, there were valid reasons to use testing very differently in order to maximize its benefits. Despite the clamor of the "experts" in the public sphere, and almost the entire media narrative pushing the opposite view, the president happened to be correct. Instead of massively testing everyone on demand, testing should be leveraged to do what *everything* should have been geared toward in the first place—protecting the high-risk, saving lives, and opening society up as soon as possible.

What was most remarkable to me from the inside was that even though the president expressed his points about testing very clearly, and many top epidemiology experts agreed, the COVID Huddles and other strategic operations were run in a different world. The messaging, the public events, the operational strategy, and the communications team pushed ahead with a focus on producing and delivering more testing to low-risk environments, schools, and communities. Reminiscent of *Catch-22*, when 150 million antigen tests became available weeks later, I was asked by several people in the COVID Huddle, "Well, now that we have these tests, what do we do with them?"

*   *   *   *   *

During my first few days, and frequently thereafter, I had my midday cookie and cappuccino with John Rader in his tiny West Wing office. Rader was my friend, but I really loved the fresh cookies from the Navy Mess just down the corridor (just kidding, John!). Rader was superbusy with many things in the administration, being a respected advisor to Kushner, but soon he would have a new responsibility—listening to my complaints and serving as a needed source of sanity. At this point, he was already a sounding board, advising me to do the most important things first. He was a voice of experience about the strong personalities in the West Wing, and a friendly face to console my frustrations.

We talked through a few of the critical issues I needed to focus on immediately. Rader fully understood the lockdowns needed to end, because people were not getting health care, families were being destroyed, kids were out of school, and the economic devastation would be incalculable. The data about the schools was overwhelming—and in my mind, there was nothing more important than opening schools. John also knew I was right that we needed to increase protections to the elderly because the chosen policies recommended by Birx and Fauci were being instituted by governors all over the country and were failing—something that was obvious from the sky-high mortality rates among seniors, but which the national press seemed reluctant to blame on either Birx and Fauci or the governors of Democratic states like New York and New Jersey. Testing was certainly one key to stopping seniors from dying, and it was also a key to safely opening schools. I told Rader what I meant by using testing to protect the elderly, and he recommended that I speak with Admiral Giroir, the person on the Task Force in charge of testing, to see what he thought about increasing tests to high-risk environments.

Of the many calls I made from Rader's office, my call about testing happened to be the first, before I even appeared at any meeting about the pandemic. I introduced myself to Giroir as the new advisor to the president. We briefly spoke. He was very friendly. He agreed with the broad reason for a discussion and suggested that he arrange a call between us two and Dr. Redfield, the director of the CDC, which was in charge of testing guidelines. Giroir arranged that immediately, and we began a conference call. I was the outsider, so I introduced myself more formally with a short summary of my background in health policy and medicine; they did the same. I remember how friendly they both were. Giroir insisted, "Scott, we are all colleagues here; please use our first names," and Dr. Redfield ("Bob") quickly agreed.

We had an informative discussion about testing—I asked questions about its rationale, its goals. I stressed my main point—that we needed to make sure the high-risk people were protected: they were dying, and this extraordinary testing capability could help with that. Nursing home residents were a special group of vulnerable Americans, not just due to their age and frailty, but also to their living situation. The evidence showed that nursing home residents had not been adequately protected; more than half of US deaths had been in assisted-living settings. I talked about priority testing of all nursing home and long-term care residents at least twice per week; testing all nursing home workers a minimum of twice per week but increasing that frequency to every day in areas with high infection activity; priority testing of all asymptomatic high-risk people with a known exposer; priority testing of all symptomatic high-risk people to protect their older social groups; proactively notifying and strictly protecting all high-risk Medicare individuals in areas of increasing community activity using COVID-like illness to the emergency rooms through ASPR; and if they were known to have been exposed, to make sure they too were tested.

I also expressed concern that people had been convinced that testing is equally urgent for everyone. That set up a misguided expectation that led to a panic among people who have no immediate need for a test but think they have to undergo one. That caused problems. When a million tests per day are conducted, that interferes with timely results from tests on priority groups. At that point in time, people were concerned about delays in receiving results; those delays meant more anxiety and resulted in quarantining many people who would days later find out they had tested negative.

Giroir and Redfield both brought up that it would be advantageous to engage people with health care knowledge in testing decisions, so that testing was done when it was needed, not just out of anxiety. We also agreed on the obvious, that a test was only valid for that single point in time and thus gave healthy people a false sense of security. Everyone agreed; we were all on the same page.

I then added what was known but never mentioned inside the White House or to my knowledge in any of the Task Force discussions—a positive test using the PCR technique in place does not necessarily mean someone is contagious. That had been well established. Fragments of dead virus hang around and can generate a positive test for many weeks or months, even though one is not generally contagious after two weeks. Moreover, PCR is extremely sensitive. It detects minute quantities of virus that do not transmit infection, if performed as it had been conducted.

This was the first of several futile attempts on my part over the next few months to generate some discussion about this hugely impactful problem—that PCR tests were the basis of defining cases, and the basis for quarantines, but most were misleading. Using a PCR "cycle threshold" of thirty-five—even lower than the thirty-seven to forty cycles used routinely to detect the virus—fewer than 3 percent of "positives" contain live, contagious virus, as reported by *Clinical Infectious Diseases*. Even the *New York Times* wrote in August that 90 percent or more of positive PCR tests falsely implied that someone was contagious. Sadly, during my entire time at the White House, this crucial fact would never even be addressed by anyone other than me at the Task Force meetings, let alone be cause for any public recommendation, even after I distributed data proving this critical point. This is just one of the many illustrations of the Task Force's inadequate consideration of scientific knowledge, an enormous indictment of the failure to assemble the necessary excellence to serve the American people in this time of crisis.

Giroir and Redfield both concluded that the testing guidelines needed to be revised. Giroir ended the call by suggesting that he would start and then circulate his draft of testing guidelines, which the Task Force would later evaluate. It was a very positive, productive, and pleasant conversation.

After the call, I was extremely upbeat. I specifically remarked to Rader, "Redfield sounded very reasonable, seems smart; he gets it." Rader burst out laughing. "That's only because he agreed with you!" I laughed, too, but it became a running joke at my expense.

*   *   *   *   *

Draft versions of testing guidelines began to circulate, beginning with Giroir and then Redfield. More than a dozen people—including those at HHS, FDA, and CDC—had provided input into what was becoming an updated guidance. All Task Force members also reviewed it; many suggested edits. The changes from the previous CDC testing guidance were visible to everyone as it circulated. It was a working document and had been passed by everyone who had the knowledge to assist. Meanwhile the vice president placed the testing guidelines on the agenda for the next Task Force meeting.

All five doctors at the table in the Situation Room—Giroir, Fauci, Birx, Redfield, and me—were directly called upon by Pence to make comments at the meeting. Giroir highlighted the most important changes, all of which had already been agreed upon by every doctor on the Task Force, as well as by others at the CDC, FDA, and HHS. Redfield and Giroir both emphasized to the group that the decision to test was now even more clearly in the hands of both the individual and their doctor—so there was now more involvement of a physician in the decision to test. That would relieve uncertainty and panic in the public and would hopefully eliminate unnecessary testing that delayed result reporting, he explained. There was also clear language stressing the critical need for frequent testing as well as protection and mitigation measures in nursing homes. First responders and those with routine contact with high-risk individuals or environments were encouraged to test frequently. Giroir also reminded everyone that there was no pullback of testing—it was better defined as who needed a test and why. All availability for testing was still there for anyone who wanted a test, he explained.

We all heard and read through these details that were placed on the desk in front of every attendee. All key changes from the current guidance on testing were highlighted. The new document provided clearer guidance for the high-risk setting of nursing homes, and guidance for general public scenarios, clarifying when certain categories of people would "not *necessarily* need a test" but should consult their doctor.

For instance, anyone exposed to an infected person but was asymptomatic, other than a high-risk person, would not "necessarily" need a test. Instead, they should consult their doctor to determine their need to get tested. Likewise, if someone had only mild symptoms, they should self-isolate and take extra precautions to protect anyone high-risk in the home; but they did not necessarily need a test, because a test would not alter treatment. Detailed instructions for handwashing, social distancing, and mask wearing were included. Explicit concerns and more stringent recommendations about testing high-risk and elderly were prominent.

Pence was very intent on making sure every doctor in the Task Force expressed their views. He virtually always asked directly for each of our comments, often by first name, and he did so in this meeting as well. All of us spoke. Birx commented on the importance of testing asymptomatic people. She argued that the only way to figure out who was sick was to test them. She memorably exclaimed, "That's why it's so dangerous—people don't even know they're sick!" I felt myself looking around the room, wondering if I was the only one who had heard this.

I commented that testing *all* asymptomatic people had a major downside—it led to confining and quarantining a massive number of healthy people with extremely low risk from COVID, and that was most of the workforce. Mass testing of low-risk people in low-risk environments was the inevitable pathway to lockdowns, and lockdowns were destructive. I reminded Birx that if people had a known exposure or lived with elderly family members, they were now recommended to ask their doctor or public health official if they should be tested. Of course, high-risk people needed protection, and I suggested that should be increased with even more frequent testing in nursing homes and other senior environments. Giroir and Redfield repeated to the entire room that this was not denying anyone a test—it was adding a doctor or a health official into the decision process. Anyway, Redfield reminded everyone that the guideline emphasized that anyone can still be tested.

Once the discussion was finished, the vice president looked around the long oval table and verified that everyone concurred. He clearly wanted to be sure he had heard all objections, which was understandable, since testing was a main focus of his Task Force, not to mention a barometer of his own achievement. Everyone—Birx, Fauci, Giroir, Redfield, and I—again agreed to the new set of guidelines.

Then someone commented that it would be improved if the language about nursing homes was moved to a specific, entirely separate section. These high-risk, vulnerable nursing home residents were a special case of vulnerable Americans. Redfield noted that nursing homes needed even more clarification than had been in previous guidelines. Everyone agreed that a call-out section would be important, especially since we wanted to reinforce the need to test nursing home staff frequently. Redfield said he and his CDC team would revise that part; they would consolidate a small section about special recommendations for nursing home testing. Pence was enthused: "Excellent work, everyone. Thank you all for your thoughtful efforts on addressing this extremely important issue. Bob, we look forward to signing off on that at the next meeting." We moved on to the next item; the VP ran a tight ship.

The next Task Force meeting also had a full agenda. As always, more items were listed than would be covered. At the end of the meeting, the VP remembered to squeeze in the testing guidance document, quickly asking for the added section on nursing homes in order to finish with the whole issue. Redfield distributed it around the table to everyone. It had no annotation of changes—all "Track Changes" indicators were now removed. I glanced through the document. It had been completely changed from the version approved by everyone at the previous Task Force meeting. True, a separate section on testing inside nursing homes had been added. However, nearly the entire document had been reverted to the original, old version of the guidance. Virtually none of the changes we had all agreed upon one week ago were present. I pulled out my notes from last week's meeting. I was correct—that entire document had been ignored.

I was stunned—I honestly thought there had been a mistake. No one else was bothering to check; they had already stood up to leave. I turned to Redfield and showed him last week's guidelines, the one we had all agreed upon after dozens of revisions. I said, "I think there's a mistake; this is not the version we all agreed on last week." He mumbled, "I just reordered a few things, that's all. Everything is there, it is just reorganized." I showed Giroir—he was confused. The VP listened to what Redfield and I were saying to each other. Pence then said he would check it out and left for his next meeting. There was no further discussion.

*   *   *   *   *

Days later, the CDC posted its new testing guidance. It was similar to what the entire Task Force had indeed agreed upon at the second-to-last meeting, along with the added nursing home guidance. It was a solid document, detailing the recommendations described by Giroir and Redfield at the Task Force, in language that was imperfect but that the general public might understand. For that brief moment, I was thinking positively about doing some good.

Almost right away, though, the pushback was on full display. The usual TV talking heads were visibly shaken, outraged, and the coverage and commentary seemed nonstop. You couldn't help but notice, because the wall-mounted TVs in nearly all offices and reception areas in the West Wing and in the EEOB, including mine, were almost always tuned to a compound array of four networks. The obsession with testing everyone, on-demand, had been undermined by the CDC. I watched and thought, "Their hair is on fire!"

As I should have anticipated, the accusations began. In the eyes of those consumed with the politics and the lockdown narrative, it could not possibly have been anything but evil forces from their nemesis, Donald Trump. Remember, only "they"—the lockdown devotees—"followed the science." And while I didn't want to believe it, everything about the pandemic was political. Emotional diatribes by CNN "medical correspondents"—with zero expertise but boiling over with conviction—went viral, as if the CDC *itself* did not create, approve, and publish this guidance. Almost immediately, CNN proclaimed with 100 percent certitude that "clearly, there had been pressure from above." The *New York Times* repeated that lie, based on pure speculation and the usual anonymous sources, blaring their misleading spin in a mendacious headline: "Top U.S. Officials Told C.D.C. to Soften Coronavirus Testing Guidelines."

Their tabloid-level attack continued with editorialized reporting to the effect that Giroir "acknowledged that the revision came after a vigorous debate among members of the White House coronavirus task force—including its newest member, Dr. Scott W. Atlas, a frequent Fox News guest and a special adviser to President Trump." As if it was inappropriate to vigorously discuss and debate every important policy question. Not to mention their bizarre implication that if I was involved, it must have been illegitimate, evil, and politically motivated.

The reality of the Washington political world took over the story. The *New York Times* wrote: "Democrats, including Speaker Nancy Pelosi and two governors—Mr. Cuomo and Gavin Newsom of California—were outraged by the changes. Mr. Newsom said California would not follow the new guidelines, and Mr. Cuomo blamed Mr. Trump. Representative Frank Pallone Jr. of New Jersey, a Democrat and the chairman of the House Energy and Commerce Committee, also chimed in on Twitter: "The Trump Admin has a lot of explaining to do." Cuomo was quoted, "We're not going to follow the CDC guidance. I consider it political propaganda."

It would have been comical if it weren't also deadly serious. These people had zero knowledge yet were overtly defiant of the authorities they used to swear by—the CDC, Fauci, and Birx. To me it was truly insane, more than just an embarrassing indictment of the entire country. These politicians are our leaders? The people in charge of the United States of America? Many friends from abroad—Switzerland, France, even Brazil—emailed me, saying, "What the hell is wrong with the United States?"

Redfield initially defended his new guidance in a written statement that was widely reported: "Everyone who needs a

COVID-19 test, can get a test. Everyone who *wants* a test does not necessarily *need* a test; the key is to engage the needed public health community in the decision with the appropriate follow-up action." The CDC Director, reassured the public that this guideline "received appropriate attention, consultation and input from task force experts." Giroir that same day held a conference call with reporters. He also defended the new testing policy and strongly denied that it arose from political pressure. "Let me tell you, right up front that the new guidelines are a CDC action," Giroir said, and noted that members of the White House coronavirus task force, including Drs. Fauci and Redfield, had discussed and agreed on the changes. I did not envy Redfield or Giroir in having to deal with this; I already knew how intent the media was on destroying people associated with this administration if they dared to defy the accepted narrative.

The heat must have been too much, though, for the more politically sensitive, image-conscious Task Force members. The first display of that was Fauci, who was quoted by Sanjay Gupta of CNN: "I was under general anesthesia in the operating room and was not part of any discussion or deliberation regarding the new testing recommendations." . And it brought home to me that I did not fit in here; in fact, I didn't want to fit in.

Honesty and integrity were still around, but it was temporary and in short supply. The same CNN reporter directly asked Giroir whether Fauci signed off on the guidelines. "Yes, all the docs signed off on this before it even got to the task force level," he replied. Giroir had personally shepherded the document around and seen its evolution, before and during the Task Force discussion. Giroir said to CNN, "I worked on them, Dr. Fauci worked on them, Dr. Birx worked on them. Dr. Hahn worked on them." The *New York Times* also reported Giroir's explanation but pounced on his subsequent inadvertent omission of Birx's name when he replied to their comments, as if it was proof that something nefarious going on. It must have been that Birx and Fauci (who claimed he was in surgery) were not even there!

A few days later, an op-ed in the *Wall Street Journal* appeared, coauthored by Stanford's Bhattacharya and Harvard's Martin Kulldorff. It was entitled, "The Case Against Covid Tests for the Young and Healthy: Hunting for asymptomatic cases encourages pointless shutdowns. Protect the vulnerable instead." These two world-class experts on viruses and testing extolled the appropriateness, the logic, the science—*the correctness*—of the new testing protocols: "The new CDC guidelines appropriately focus testing resources on hospital workers and the older generation.... With the new CDC guidelines, strategic age-targeted viral testing will protect older people from deadly Covid-19 exposure and children and young adults from needless school closures."

Once again, the media's claim "all experts agreed" that the CDC guidelines were wrong was a lie. The assertion that all experts agreed with the lockdowns, the mass testing, school closures, and other measures implemented all over the country—measures that had failed while being pushed by Birx, Fauci, and the mainstream media—was also a lie.

The media was rabid. Anonymous "officials" were quoted saying that the document was "published against scientists' objections"—as if the scientists they always trusted, Fauci, Birx, the CDC, HHS, and the FDA, had not all approved and written it; as if the director of the CDC himself had not written, finalized, and then published the document himself. The blame was directed against HHS officials or me or the president—anyone except Fauci and Birx—because it simply had to be that way. An unending stream of wild accusations and smears filled the media, all from people who knew nothing about the truth. Pure speculation was published and repeated endlessly as fact.

What happened next was another "Welcome to Washington" moment.

Suddenly, after that two-week flurry of media hit pieces, politically filled accusations, and a full-throttle takedown by many public health organizations, a new testing guidance popped up on the CDC website. No discussion at the Task Force. No explanation given. No request for input from others with knowledge about such a complex and impactful issue. And it reflected a *180-degree reversal* of the revision of two weeks earlier. This CDC document simply reiterated its old testing guidelines. It now comported with what was demanded by the media, by the on-the-record purveyors pushing the lockdowns and the massive testing narrative.

I asked Redfield what had happened—I knew it would come up in the next press briefing, and I would be the one stuck with explaining his agency's actions to what was already an outrageously hostile, vicious media. He replied with some unintelligible explanation trying to trivialize the change and then offhandedly remarked that "he and the Ambassador discussed it and revised it."

At first, I didn't know who the hell he was talking about. Then I remembered the penchant for titles among bureaucrats. "The Ambassador" referred to Birx from her days in the Obama administration. Politics and media pressure had prevailed, science and logic be damned. What really mattered to some of these Task Force doctors was public perception in the media. To me, that was a disgrace. I again asked myself, "What am I doing here?"

CHAPTER 6
My Role as the President's Advisor

Expressing his opinion about the Task Force members to CNN on September 27, 2020, Dr. Anthony Fauci remarked, "Most are working together. I think, you know, what the outlier is."

I was proud to be the outlier in this group—and not just because I was totally right, while the "inliers" were disastrously wrong. My personal character and background also make me an outlier, particularly among the Washington political class and academic elites.

Feisty independence and blunt talk run deep in my family roots. My grandparents arrived in America in the early 1900s through Ellis Island. They came with nothing, and they survived on their own determination, hard work, and grit. My mother's mother, a tenaciously independent woman, taught me many lessons, but one frequent injunction stands out: "Become educated!" she repeated over and over again, because she was not.

My father was a "free spirit" who chose his own path—he answered to himself and no one else. He enlisted in the Marines, after Pearl Harbor. He came back without the patience for college, so he began a life of work. He chose jobs that allowed him personal freedom—salesman, taxi driver, hair stylist—and lived paycheck to paycheck at best. After finishing high school and marrying at nineteen, my mother worked full-time as a secretary for her entire career while raising me and my brother.

I was raised in the Midwest, in a small, attached townhouse alongside the interstate highway on-ramp in a lower-income part of a middle-class suburb. My parents squeaked by. They were proud of me, but top grades were not even close to sufficient. I wasn't putting out enough effort as a student, and that was worrisome to them. It mattered to try much harder, to achieve to the absolute best of my abilities. The point of that took me many years to realize.

My brother and I were the first in our family to attend college. Along the way, I worked in odd jobs—busboy, roach exterminator, pizza deliverer, post office mail sorter—throughout high school and college. It wasn't just to pay for school; my dad needed that money to pay our family's bills. My jobs in college and medical school supplemented scholarships and loans, but I ultimately came out of medical school from the University of Chicago under a mountain of debt. That didn't matter. I was proud to have done it on my own. No one paid for my education, because my family had no money. No one manipulated the system to get me accepted, because I had no connections. No one paved my way. But my parents did give me the most important thing a child could have. I was treated as if I mattered. I was taught to speak my mind, to question authority, and to never be afraid to say what I knew is true. No matter what.

These habits soon began to pay off. I was named chief resident at Northwestern University and worked extremely long hours to excel as a neuroradiology fellow at the University of Pennsylvania. I later joined that department as an assistant professor to augment the world's best neuroradiology group. Neuroradiology entails integrating advanced medical imaging with complex information from multiple subspecialties—neurology, cardiology, infectious disease, oncology, pediatrics, neurosurgery, orthopedics, ophthalmology, and all the rest—in arriving at a diagnosis and then advising on the best course of action. As an educator, I didn't bother detailing lists of possible diagnoses, like most other professors. The difference between a great diagnostician and a good one is not the amount you can memorize. Instead, I taught how to sort out a mass of complicated information and use logic to deduce the correct diagnosis. I also told my trainees something else: "If you know the diagnosis, then just say it! Don't be afraid—when you're right, you're right. *Period.*"

With others contributing, I wrote and edited what became a standard book in a revolutionary field, *MRI of the Brain and Spine*, starting it before I even finished my training. While a faculty member at the nation's top medical centers, I worked in patient care, conducted research, and trained more than one hundred of the next leaders in neuroradiology and MRI. I was honored to be a visiting professor at almost every top medical school in the country and an invited speaker all over the world, with honors and accolades from inside and outside the United States.

In my first few years at Stanford in the early 2000s, a new challenge arose—health care system reform. I quickly realized that the discussion was being dominated by health economists. They looked at incentives, financial models, and spreadsheets, without the perspective of a doctor who understood the complexities of patient care. As accomplished and smart as they were, almost none had a real understanding of the value of medical technology and subspecialty health care. They didn't have an understanding of the value of sophisticated diagnostics, minimally invasive treatments, and what matters most to save sick patients.

After fourteen years as professor and chief of neuroradiology at Stanford to top off my twenty-five years in academic medicine as a professor, teacher, clinician, and researcher, I decided to make a complete shift to health care policy. After a decade juggling two faculty jobs with two offices at Stanford, one in the medical school and one at the Hoover Institution, I finally accepted a full-time, endowed position in health policy at Hoover.

For seventeen years, I have worked in health policy, still learning so much from the world's best economists and policy scholars. My colleagues can count on me for two consistencies. First, my presentations include too many slides detailing facts—graphs, charts, statistical comparisons—sometimes to the point of boredom, and always generating a reminder to "wrap it up." Second, when I speak, I speak directly and candidly. After she was appointed as the new director of Hoover, Condi Rice called me into her office. She wanted to learn the nuances of what she was about to encounter from us faculty members. Why ask me? Condi told me, "Scott, you are my truth teller."

Throughout my career, my approach to questions has also remained constant, no matter where I have been. If I don't know an answer, I say, "I don't know." But then I make sure to figure it out. I focus on knowing the data *in detail*. And in my work, I judge people on that basis—what they know and how hard they work to know it. I am not impressed with someone's boarding school or Ivy League diploma. And I never assume that any title, credential, or any amount of wealth necessarily confers superior knowledge. Personal accomplishment—my record—is the measure, not the university crest on my parking sticker.

But I never understood how much of an outlier I was until I entered the world of Washington, DC, in August 2020 to advise the president of the United States. Before I arrived, I frankly did not have much respect for most politicians. They inhabit a world where truth doesn't necessarily take precedence, where glad-handing and *quid pro quo* relationships are the currency of the day, instead of knowledge and critical thinking. That's not me. I am not a political person. I am not a schmoozer.

Being an outlier also meant that my motivation as an advisor to the president was different. I came to Washington in spite of the politics, not because of them. I wasn't interested in working in Washington or positioning myself for something bigger. I didn't come to the White House to make friends or mingle with the politically powerful. I thought the advice coming out of the Task Force doctors was horribly off base, and I wanted to stop the harms from both the virus and the lockdown policies. My statements and advice were never adjusted to back up the president. I came there to tell him what *I* thought, not to be a mouthpiece for what *he* thought. I came there to speak on behalf of the American public, especially those who were being destroyed by the lockdowns. And I could not sit silent and watch this mass destruction.

That singular motivation made me an outlier on the Task Force too. The other doctors there had other motivations. That's not to say they didn't want to end the pandemic and help the country, but they had additional pressures. Some on the Task Force and in the health agencies were undoubtedly influenced by political considerations. They had government careers to worry about. They had "relationships" in the health agencies and influential friends to please in the media.

And there was one other difference—none were health policy researchers. There was no health policy scholar on the Task Force before I arrived. There were, however, proven "survivors" of previous political administrations. That does not imply neutrality at all—it implies an insider's knowledge of how to successfully align with other career bureaucrats to gain political allies. Surviving for that many years underscores the strength and success of those alliances, absolutely crucial to navigating such an environment. That's how it works in Washington, I learned.

*　*　*　*　*

Despite how foreign Washington felt to me throughout my four months there, after a few days, every day had some sameness. I relocated to the Trump Hotel from the Willard after a short time, because the Willard couldn't book me continually due to a prior sellout. I did not know my future, but I could not deal with the hassle of moving out and then back in. I walked out of the White House security gates at Pennsylvania Avenue one evening and headed to the Trump Hotel to check it out. They had no idea who I was—perfect, I wanted to be anonymous—and I was shown the possible rooms for what I said could be anywhere from a couple of weeks to a few months. The one thing that impressed me was their security setup, where even approaching the front entrance required clearance.

My days began by passing through an initial set of gates at the security entrance just past the Treasury Building. I was always impressed by the friendliness and professionalism of the agents stationed there, actually everywhere inside the White House and its grounds. The beauty and tranquility inside the secure area were a stark contrast to the reality of my time in Washington. On my left was the Department of Treasury, straight ahead the Washington Monument, and on my right, I could peer through the gates toward the White House and a bit of the North Lawn.

After I was screened through the final entrance, I almost always entered through the grand East Wing doors, saying good morning to the agent at the desk, then continuing inside through the ground floor of the residential part of the White House, passing next to the legendary Rose Garden, and eventually emerging inside the West Wing.

This walk was always impressive, amazing every single day; I never took it for granted. It was not simply walking by the historic paintings of first ladies or the legendary rooms where heads of state were entertained or even seeing the Rose Garden, smaller than expected and nearly always being tended to by a crew. To me, it was the photographs in the corridor, filled with decades of historic scenes of presidents and first ladies with visiting dignitaries or with their famous pets, often on the South Lawn or in the Oval Office. I often thought it was a shame most Americans would never experience the special feeling of entering that building or viewing up-close the White House, the South and North Lawns. I had never seriously reflected on being an American, but I could not help feeling awed by it all, surprised every morning by my own sense of patriotism as I entered the East Wing.

Occasionally, I would walk outside instead, alongside the White House, through the kitchen service areas toward EEOB. When I chose that route, I would emerge from the protected passageway outside the James S. Brady Press Briefing Room. To the right, the broadcast media tents for interviews and a set of standing microphones were stationed near the North Lawn for the press gaggles later that day. Eventually, I learned to hold my White House badge in my hand as I passed by on my way to the EEOB, since the Secret Service guards were very serious about who was permitted in that area. I was glad, especially later, when we had the scare about the shooter during the president's press briefing.

* * * * *

I soon began to appreciate the terrain inside the White House and therefore what my role would encompass. Two parallel worlds concerning the pandemic existed in the administration, and these worlds were in direct opposition to each other. On one hand, the president had identified, by his own common sense, what was patently obvious. It made no sense to suddenly shut down the entire American economy, essentially lock everyone up, for a virus that was severely dangerous only to the elderly and others with significant underlying diseases. He had no list of facts, but it wasn't hard to see that the lockdowns, if they continued, were going to be extremely destructive. The booming economy, the key to America's domestic strength and international power, as well as the administration's main accomplishment, would disappear, with massive job loss. He also grasped the obvious, as would every parent, that children should be in school. If kids were not in school, it meant their parents could not work. And despite all the smart people around the president, no one ever mentioned the most obvious fact of all: the lockdowns were failing to prevent old people from dying, even though it was known from day one who the most vulnerable people were.

On the other hand, his own administration's public health experts on the VP's Task Force were putting forward recommendations that promoted the very strategy he opposed: restricting business operations, testing and quarantining healthy people, closing schools, reducing group sizes, limiting travel and family gatherings. And those contradictory recommendations were not just presented in the media and to the public. All internal meetings involving Birx were filled with warnings and exhortations advocating locking society down, although never using those words. The medical recommendations in the Task Force meetings, run by the VP, focused only on stopping the virus and never once cautioned about the health impacts of closures and confinements.

The three-times weekly COVID Huddles for planning White House communications were run by Kushner and typically included the president's highest-level advisors on communications, including Hope Hicks, as well as many other administration spokespeople frequently interviewed in the media. In those meetings, virtually the entire communications and events team, aside from Kayleigh McEnany, who never attended, was hearing that same viewpoint straight from Dr. Birx. There was a baffling dissonance between the stated policies of the president, known to everyone in the room, and the output from his administration's communications.

I was there to help inform the administration's pandemic policy, including proposing ways to highlight those principles to the public. However, much to my frustration, I was often the lone voice making the internal case, including to the communications group, that the lockdowns were incorrect. The elderly were dying, the virus was not stopped from spreading, and the lockdowns were inflicting massive harms. Moreover, the data that formed the basis of understanding by these nonmedical people and guided their communications was being misinterpreted. My task was to inform everyone internally, but that was extremely challenging, because it meant I had to disagree with Dr. Birx, on the most fundamental points, in her presence, to the group that had come to rely totally on her for months.

The second, and in my mind far more consequential, aspect of my role was speaking the truth to the American people. That would be done directly via my own interviews and writings, and indirectly through the president. I was there to help the president understand the pandemic, which included updating him on ongoing research and adding another voice to advise him about the facts as more was learned. This was the real reason I had come. For his prepared remarks on the pandemic, my job was to provide additional input and to translate the science into policy that he could communicate. Those drafting his briefings, people like Stephen Miller, Derek Lyons, and other influential insiders like Hope Hicks and Kayleigh, believed in his views about protecting the elderly and opening up the economy; they agreed with my views on the pandemic and the harms of the lockdowns.

I also stood ready in the president's press conferences, available to answer questions at his discretion, to clarify remarks, but most significantly to speak from that extraordinarily visible platform directly to the American people. That part of my job had nothing to do with the Task Force, nothing to do with convincing Birx or Fauci, and nothing to do with the media who were engaged in their own self-important battles. I viewed my responsibility as being purely to the president and the American people and no one else. And I took that responsibility more seriously than anything else in my life.

Each time the president decided to hold a press conference in the Brady Press Room, I was asked for my involvement in two ways. First, the remarks to be read by the president were circulated for input from several people. I was requested to provide and verify certain data points, add anything I thought would be important for him to mention, and edit or validate other people's inputs. That required my 24/7 availability, very quick replies, and 100 percent verifiable sources.

Once those remarks were finalized by the staff sec and Stephen Miller, a small group of people gathered in the Oval Office, right before the press conference. During those pre-briefings, the president would go through the prepared remarks as he sat behind the *Resolute* Desk, black marker in hand. If he had any questions related to the pandemic, he would turn to me. At times, I would offer up something I thought he needed to understand, even if I wasn't asked. Others would speak up on different topics or voice additional guidance, particularly updating him to be ready for certain topics that had become newsworthy that day.

None of my advice was geared toward a political end. Before I arrived, the most influential faces of public health were filling the void left since he had discontinued the pandemic press with their own interviews, and they added to the public's uncertainty, creating more fear through their comments. The president, I recommended, must lead visibly, speak personally, because the panic itself was dangerous and leading to the propagation of harmful policies across the states.

Americans desperately needed to feel this president was knowledgeable and closely monitoring the situation. I advised that the president himself should be presenting data, including numbers, trends, and specific updates. That should include setting expectations and providing perspective—for instance, noting that cases would increase with more social mingling, that infections among high-risk individuals were far more problematic than the total number of positive tests, and even that hospitalizations and some deaths would certainly follow, despite our best efforts.

Fear of the unknown was paralyzing America, and the media was inciting even more panic by sensationalizing any increases in cases or deaths as if those were always preventable or unexpected, or occurring uniquely in the US due to mismanagement. Meanwhile, the public needed to hear that progress was proceeding rapidly on drugs and vaccines, including specific time lines. Even though details were not his style and he had not spoken about data beforehand, I believed it would be most reassuring if the president himself delivered that level of information.

I also felt it wasn't good enough to warn people ad nauseam to "wash their hands, use social distancing, avoid crowds, and wear masks when appropriate." Yes, it was important, and I made sure those key recommendations were included in every single briefing, every speech, and every update the president issued. That said, we all knew the president had his own style. He loved to wander off script and without fail he would speak off the top of his head no matter what was in front of him.

Instead of simply admonishing people for the thousandth time about what everyone already knew, he also needed to emphasize *how* to protect the elderly, to include more specifics about increasing the protection of those at highest risk. Using their standard mitigation measures and the lockdowns that were in place almost everywhere, the elderly were not being protected sufficiently. I wanted the president to stress the three foundations of a more targeted strategy: more diligently protecting the most vulnerable; mobilizing resources to avoid hospital overcrowding; and safely opening schools and society.

To back up those words, I pushed internally for an even more intense focus on increasing protection of those vulnerable Americans. That included far more frequent testing in high-risk settings, tying increased testing of long-term care staff to community illness trends, and sending millions of new, rapid tests to nonresidential senior centers and historically Black colleges. Working with Seema Verma, the administrator of CMS, along with Brad Smith of the domestic policy staff, we succeeded in prioritizing those policies throughout my time there. If the president would only articulate those extra protections in his remarks, I contended, it would help mitigate the anxiety that we were helpless against the virus.

It was most critical, in my view, that the president provide clearer justification for reopening society. He needed to make the case that the lockdown was killing people by interfering with important medical care, destroying families, and sacrificing children. Economists (and all competent public health experts) have long understood that unemployment, job losses, and economic devastation itself directly *caused* major physical and psychological health harms, drug abuse, child abuse, and even loss of lives. The president needed to stress these facts, not just allow the fear-addicted media and power-hungry lockdown advocates to perpetuate the myth that there was a stark choice between saving the economy and saving lives.

In almost every briefing or speech from August onwards, the president provided specific data updating the public on trends in problematic parts of the country; he reminded people to use the standard cautionary measures; he stressed the importance of opening schools and society while diligently protecting the elderly; he put into perspective how the entire world was struggling to limit the damage from the pandemic; and he stated very directly something that almost no one seemed to understand, including several on the White House Task Force—that locking down society would not eliminate or stamp out the virus

* * * * *

I soon came to feel that walking into the Brady Press Room was like entering into a battle, one that I profoundly disliked. I had no interest in what I viewed as a totally unprofessional session filled with vulgar hostility from most of the reporters in the room. The sole aim of most in that room was to do combat, to disagree, to put you on the defensive. The beauty of it was that they actually knew so little that it was like dealing with an argumentative teenager; that didn't make it pleasant though.

Nonetheless, it always amazed me that the president seemed to feel very differently. No matter what was on the agenda, regardless of the shouting and whatever ignorant, accusatory questions were thrown at him, he clearly enjoyed the interaction. Perhaps he knew that he would win by simply driving the reporters crazy. Faced with demands for certain responses they thought were impossible to deny, he would never provide those responses, if only to frustrate their expectations. I always felt that if a reporter had told him to admit that one plus one equaled two, he would simply refuse—just because.

On one occasion, after the usual Oval Office pre-briefing and run-through of the script and pertinent issues to be covered, Kayleigh showed the president the day's new seating chart.

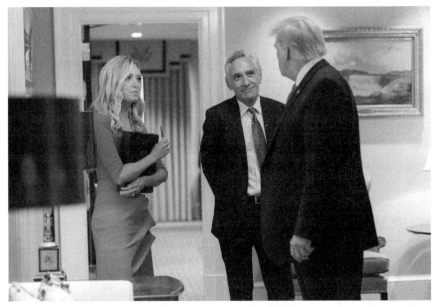

Standing just outside of the Oval Office, Kayleigh McEnany and I had a private conversation about the press briefing with President Trump. (*Credit: Official White House photographers*)

She pointed out two reporters in particular who would likely be hostile. I took that as her way of alerting him that their questions would be notably unfair. More likely, they would drop all pretense of asking legitimate questions and just go into full-blown accusation mode. I had already seen that happen more than once. Although it was a shock the first time, it became normal to hear reporters bark out angrily, "When will you stop lying to the American people?!" or shout, "You killed hundreds of thousands of Americans!" as he walked out after the conference.

President Trump listened and nodded, as if he would heed her warning. Then he said energetically, "OK, let's go!" Kayleigh and I entered the room first, sat to the side of the podium, and awaited the president's entrance, as was customary. When the president entered, we all stood, and he began by reading his prepared remarks. As always, the president ad-libbed as he covered most if not all of the remarks in his folder, at times glancing over to me and casually commenting. He then closed his folder, looked up, and began to call on the assembled reporters.

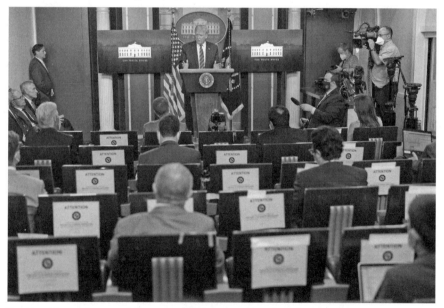

President Trump dominated the press conferene as I sat in a chair alongside Larry Kudlow and Secretary Steve Mnuchin, ready for questions. (Credit: Official White House photographers)

To my surprise, President Trump immediately pointed directly at the first reporter Kayleigh had warned him to skip. The reporter asked some forgettable question, and the president answered it aggressively, denying the premise. Next, he pointed directly at the second reporter "to be avoided" and did the same. It was classic Trump.

I sat there laughing, realizing that he had no fear whatsoever. He knew he controlled the room. No one could possibly intimidate him. In retrospect, I should have expected it.

Soon after I became a part of these regular briefings, the reality of being inside the White House alongside the president came home to me in a totally unanticipated way. In this early August briefing, I sat to the president's right, in one of the chairs adjacent to the stage. This time, Secretary Mnuchin and Acting Director of the Office of Management and Budget Russ Vought occupied the other chairs next to me. This briefing would include a discussion of the economy, so I figured Mnuchin and Vought would be answering most of the questions. The briefing began in the usual way, with the president at the podium reading from his prepared remarks. But he was suddenly interrupted by an entering Secret Service security agent, who discreetly told him to exit. After the president was escorted out, we all followed, knowing nothing about why.

Entering the foyer and office area just outside the briefing room, we encountered a group of heavily armed men, what looked like SWAT teams, weapons in hand. Several other agents, presumably Secret Service, were also there, along with the usual staffers behind them, standing outside their small offices. The atmosphere felt tense, not chaotic but sort of disorienting.

I was standing a few feet from the president. Our eyes turned to the sets of television monitors right outside the press briefing room, already reporting on the abrupt interruption. I listened as the president asked for more details about what was happening; we all kept one eye glued to the TV coverage. Apparently, there was a shooter nearby, but it was stressed that he was outside the White House grounds. There had been gunshots, someone said, but beyond the barrier fence. Someone commented to the president, asking if he was all right. The president glanced around and said, "Of course, look around, there could be nowhere safer," pointing out the impressive security throng that had so swiftly arrived to protect him. I was pretty relieved myself, paradoxically feeling safer to be standing right there.

Several minutes passed as we all watched the reporting on the TVs. After some time, we were cleared to reenter the briefing room. President Trump said, "OK, let's go," and we all walked back into the room with the president leading the way. He took the stage, standing behind the podium, ready to resume as if nothing unusual had happened. I couldn't help but notice that the reporters looked scared, even behind their masks, frequently glancing toward the wall of windows. It was a vivid contrast to the president, who calmly carried on despite knowing that he was the likely target of a gunman. Reporters called out several questions about how he felt to come back in, should he continue, was he frightened, what had happened—but it was they who seemed frightened silly.

*   *   *   *   *

As part of my role I was frequently called to the Oval Office to provide updates on the pandemic or to give my opinions and answer questions on various topics. The point was to answer the president's questions, help him think through certain elements of the evolving situation, or anticipate and help him prepare for questions in his frequent press conferences, interviews, or special events.

Same-day COVID testing was required for all who would see the president or VP that day. That meant I would be tested, without fail, in the EEOB facility that morning, if I would later be entering the Oval Office or attending a Task Force meeting. Since I did not arrive until the end of July, the simpler, more comfortable rapid tests were already available. Obviously, testing has its limits, but it was an important part of the West Wing protocol.

There was never any certainty about what questions I would be asked. Regardless of the reason for a briefing, a variety of topics always came up, one question leading to another. These conversations were very direct, without small talk, and there was a free exchange of thoughts. If the president asked me a question, I gave him my unvarnished opinion. There was never any filter on the president, nor was there a filter on me. I made sure I was prepared, but if I did not know something, I never spoke as if I did. This was way too important to pretend otherwise. I was very blunt from the start—I would never agree with something that was not true, no matter who said it. I would never have remained silent in front of the American people when the president brought up drinking disinfectant at a press conference. Nor would I have done so when unproven recommendations about treatments were put forth. Then again, I was not a career bureaucrat.

At only one or two of the Oval Office briefings I attended in early August, Dr. Birx and I were both present to answer questions or clarify certain points for the president. Occasionally, the key people involved in Operation Warp Speed were also called in—Dr. Slaoui, Secretary Azar, Paul Mango of HHS, or General Perna, for instance.

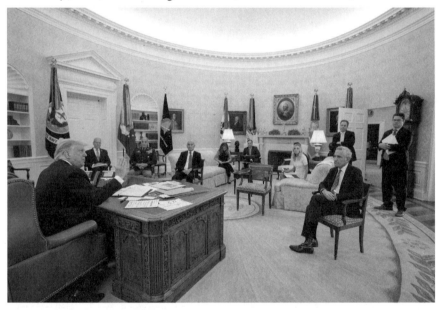

In the Oval Office, I sat in the arc of chairs in front of President Trump with HHS Advisor Paul Mango (far left), General Gus Perna (center), and Moncef Slaoui (center)—three key members of Operation Warp Speed, while President Trump held court. Kayleigh McEnany (seated), Derek Lyons (standing near door), and other key advisors listened. (*Credit: Official White House photographers*)

After my initial few weeks as advisor, though, I never saw Birx again in the Oval Office. Fauci was never present. That was a big change for both Fauci and Birx, because in the early months they were regularly seen alongside the president in the press conferences. That meant they were certainly in the pre-briefings, too, even though all of the so-called Task Force press conferences had stopped quite a while before I arrived.

One memorable pre-briefing during August proceeded with both Birx and me seated in front of the president, in the arc of four or five chairs arranged in front of his desk. As usual, close to a half dozen more people were further behind me, seated on the sofas or standing, but I don't remember who was in the room.

To no one's surprise, the president brought up one of his favorite topics—testing. By then, he and I had discussed testing several times—not just the massive testing apparatus that had been developed, and not just his frustrations at having "cases" defined by a test, even if a person is not sick. We had gone over the importance of frequent testing in protecting high-risk individuals, its impact on the safety of health care workers, and its pitfalls in keeping schools and businesses open. Testing was a complex policy topic, far more complicated and nuanced than the "test, test, test" mantra voiced endlessly by almost everyone in the media. It was a critical tool that had significant value when used properly.

We went through the importance of leveraging the massive testing capacity to save lives. The importance of increasing testing in nursing home staff and the elderly was emphasized. Testing to protect the people who had a significant risk from the virus was the most important point. Testing was very important in all high-risk environments, especially in hospitals and patient care settings. We also discussed how testing should be used to help open society safely, rather than be used to quarantine low-risk, healthy people and shut down the lowest-risk environments like schools. Toward the end of this Oval Office pre-briefing, the president asked Birx directly, "Do you agree with Scott on the testing?"

I knew where Birx stood on the issue. Testing had also already been a topic in the Task Force meetings, although that discussion was not fully fleshed out. I looked to my right, where she sat, as she began adjusting her position in her chair. She hesitantly replied, "Yes, I think so," and she looked at me for affirmation. I was emotionless, but her half-hearted statement was a lie. I think the president probably sensed that, so he turned his eyes toward me and asked me, "Scott, is that true?"

Without hesitating, I answered his question. "No, she doesn't agree. Dr. Birx thinks we should be testing healthy, asymptomatic people, and if they are positive, they need to be quarantined for fourteen days. And even if exposed people test negative, they still need to be quarantined." I matter-of-factly went on, eyes straight ahead looking at the president. "And that leads to locking down healthy, low-risk people, and those are the people that make up the workforce. That leads to locking down businesses and closing schools." The president nodded but said nothing.

Since this was the last of many topics covered in this pre-briefing, the president ended the discussion and walked into the room connected to the Oval Office.

We all stood to leave. It felt very tense, but there was zero chance I would lie to the president of the United States. He asked me a direct question, and I answered it truthfully. There was no dilemma, no choice in my mind. Birx apparently felt otherwise. She threw a fit, right there, in front of everyone, as we stood near the door before leaving the Oval Office. She was furious, screaming at me, "NEVER DO THAT AGAIN!! AND IN THE OVAL!!"

I felt pretty bad, because she was so angry. I had absolutely no desire for conflict. But did she actually expect me to lie to the president, just to cover up for her? I responded, "Sorry, but he asked me a question, so I answered it." I glanced at a couple of others in the room who had seen the entire episode and muttered, "Well, that didn't go very well," as I exited.

CHAPTER 7
Meet the Press!

I was working at a frantic pace, multitasking as best I could. Because I treated every request as urgent, real-time, I felt added pressure; but nothing was more urgent than vetting the president's public remarks. Adding to the requirement for my input was that this president loved engaging with the press. That meant that a new briefing could be called at any moment, and those briefings were frequent. I came to assume that there would be a press briefing every day, and for every briefing, there would be a pandemic update. I was one of many who were asked for input—topics, data, edits, sources of numbers, trends, and anything I thought would be important to highlight or include, thematically or otherwise. It was not simply the magnitude of the pandemic that created my concerns, it was the requirement for perfect accuracy in every detail.

Despite my initial involvement, Kushner had kept to his desire to shield me from what he knew would be an assault by the media; we had no immediate plan to change that approach. But this was not a highly structured environment. My unveiling to the press by the president was spur-of-the-moment, totally unplanned.

In the first several days after my arrival, I was not yet involved in the "pre-briefing" that occurred just before the president entered the Brady Press Briefing room to deliver his remarks. A small but varying group of relevant advisors would join the president in the Oval Office. He would sit behind the *Resolute* Desk, going through the printout handed to him by the staff sec. Usually, Kayleigh, Stephen Miller, Kushner, Derek Lyons, Hope Hicks, and a few others would stand or sit as the president looked through and hand-edited what he wanted to use as his script. As he sat with his marker deleting or adding specific points, he would ask questions to those in the Oval Office about particular issues. At times, people would also offer comments they thought he should hear, even if he didn't ask. I soon became a fixture in those pre-briefings. But in the beginning, I was inputting remarks beforehand, via the staff sec's creation and editing process.

On this day, after I finished my inputs and others had finalized them, the printouts were brought up to the president. I spontaneously decided to go up to Kayleigh's office to show her some data and explain some important points about various trends. This was something I often did, because I wanted to make sure that Kayleigh fully understood not just the statements themselves, but the data behind them, so she would be fully armed for the inevitable pushback from the press.

This time, Kayleigh was standing at her desk. She showed me the final edit of what would be said in minutes to the nation by the president. I froze—the editing process had created a small change that in turn generated an incorrect statement about the pandemic data. That was my domain, and I absolutely could not let the president state something that was not 100 percent correct. I nervously told Kayleigh this must be corrected. She quickly said, "We better go in to tell him, right now; he's about to give the briefing."

We hustled over to the Oval Office. As we entered the anteroom, Kushner was standing at the doorway, and I quickly explained there was an error in the remarks. He gestured to me, saying, "OK, go in there and tell him." The president was already standing, beginning to exit the Oval Office, talking as he headed toward the doorway. I spoke up.

"Excuse me, Mr. President."

"Hi, Scott!" he smiled broadly, with his booklet of remarks in hand.

"There is a mistake in your remarks," I declared.

He stopped in his tracks. "What mistake?"

"The sentence in there now says 'with no increase in deaths' but it should say 'with no significant increase in deaths.' That's not the same thing."

President Trump looked around, seemingly surprised that I would care about this trivial detail. I was uncertain what would come next. He then announced to the small group walking with him, "If this were anyone else, I wouldn't change it. But since Scott says it should be changed, then I will." With that, he took out his marker, made the change, and flipped me the pen to keep. I smiled, said thanks, and then he continued to walk toward the briefing room.

Unexpectedly, he turned to look over his shoulder. "Scott, want to come in with me?" Kushner and I looked at each other. We both knew this would alter the plan of my remaining in the background. I instinctively said, "OK, sure," and we began walking. Jared smiled, shrugged his shoulders, and said, "OK, well, here goes. Good luck!"

The president, Kayleigh, and I walked toward the entrance. I nervously turned to Kayleigh. "Kayleigh, please tell me exactly where to go, exactly where to sit, exactly what to do!" Smiling at my anxiety, she instructed me to enter first, before her, and sit in the far chair on the side. So I did.

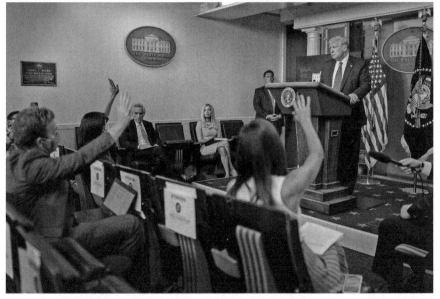

In my first appearance in the Brady Press Room, the President entertained questions while I watched alongside Kayleigh McEnany. *(Credit: Official White House photographers)*

And for that briefing, all I could do was sit there and try to come up with something, just in case the president asked, as he often did, if I "wanted to say a few words."

That didn't happen, and I was relieved. However, my unveiling in the Briefing Room was handled very awkwardly, with only an offhanded comment from the president at the podium. "Everyone knows Scott Atlas, right? Scott is a very famous man, who is also highly respected," President Trump said. "He's working with us and will be working with us on the coronavirus. And he has many great ideas."

Instead of explaining my background as a health policy expert of more than fifteen years with an extensive medical background, it was left to the press to define me. And of course, they did. That lack of preparedness by the White House communications team was harmful to me and the president himself.

This episode foreshadowed many shocks about the workings of the White House. I assumed that everyone in the West Wing would understand that if the special advisor to the president was attacked, it undermined the president's own credibility. Of course, that was the intent of the attackers, which is why it continues even today. At the very least, I had anticipated that the White House would be on solid footing in terms of dealing with a hostile press. I expected a highly skilled, coordinated group that knew how to push back on "fake news," because that seemed to be a constant in Washington.

I could not have been more wrong. Not only was there no polished, professional team prepared for dealings with the press, it was if there was no previous experience with such dealings. Kayleigh herself was absolutely outstanding—she knew her stuff cold, and her preparation on a huge portfolio of issues was truly amazing. I was constantly in awe of her poise but even more at her total mastery of the material.

Other than Kayleigh, though, the White House communications team was amateurish at best. To my knowledge, they reported to Chief of Staff Mark Meadows. With one or two exceptions, the team was a group of young people, very nice, but in way over their heads. That left it up to me to defend my own credibility and to fight the discrediting of the president's remarks on the pandemic.

Without the unforgettable support of two extraordinary, truly exceptional people—the phenomenal Liz Horning, senior advisor to the Counsel to the President, and (outside Washington) a brilliant senior advisor to a prominent governor—I would have been almost totally on my own.

* * * * *

The pandemic had been an ongoing nightmare for eight months before I set foot in DC. In my eyes, the administration was in total disarray. They were sending out two contrary messages: the Task Force was pushing the Birx-Fauci lockdowns, while at the same time, the president was pushing for reopening. This conflict was not only chaotic; it was highlighted by the anti-Trump media. That created fear and uncertainty in the population. And through it all, hundreds of thousands of people were dying, despite the lockdowns. Yes, the elites—including the political class, the media, and professionals able to work from home—were inconvenienced, no doubt. But the bulk of the country, especially working class and poor families, was being destroyed by the closures and shutdowns.

On top of this gross failure of public health leadership, the media constantly threw gasoline on the fire by highlighting every negative about the pandemic, even when positive news was available. No opportunity to inflame the voters was going to be missed by what I now believe are the most despicable group of unprincipled liars one could ever imagine—the American media.

No question, the Trump administration's communications team was overwhelmed; so perhaps I should have anticipated that they would also be unprepared for my casual introduction to the media. I was naive, though. I assumed the White House team understood that if I was delegitimized, then the president would be undermined as well. They certainly should have had enough experience by now to understand the need to present adequate credentials for presidential appointments. Clearly my assumptions were wrong. But even after witnessing their amateurish bungling in allowing a hostile media to define me, I was still not prepared for what happened.

An all-out attempt to undermine my credibility was immediately underway, involving gross distortions, straw man arguments based on blatant misrepresentations of my views, and straight-out lies. First, my background. I had been a health policy scholar for more than fifteen years, in an endowed senior faculty position at one of the most respected policy institutes in the world. Several years earlier, in 2012, I had pivoted from medicine to a focus on health policy, resigning from my faculty position as professor and chief of neuroradiology at Stanford University Medical Center. This career shift was accomplished after nearly three decades as a professor at America's finest medical centers from coast to coast, twenty-five years in academic medicine at the very top of my field. I was an honorary member of several medical societies, a visiting professor all over the world and at nearly every major academic medical center in the country, a sought-after speaker who had written several acclaimed books, and a policy expert who had recently testified to Congress about the pandemic. I had never bothered to mention my academic background in public, let alone to anyone in the West Wing, because to me it was self-evident and frankly undignified.

None of that mattered. The media refused to be truthful about my background, engaging in propaganda tactics scarcely different from those used by regimes like the USSR or Communist China to discredit political enemies. Everyone had warned me that anyone willing to stand next to the president was going to be attacked, but the vitriol still threw me. It was not that I expected fairness. But I was not prepared for the total lack of integrity and even basic decency in America's media. Willful distortion and lies to destroy anyone willing to answer the president's call to help the country were now totally acceptable.

At one point, I walked into Rader's office, shaking my head. "John," I said, "I don't think they know who I am. They don't understand that this is not at all a political position."

John looked at me with uncharacteristic intensity; his usual easygoing smile had disappeared. Having been in Washington for several years by then, he immediately set me straight. "No, Scott, *you* are the one who doesn't understand. The moment you were introduced in that room, you became part of this administration."

I was completely taken aback. I absolutely did not understand that, not one bit. None of my motivation for being there was political. What the hell was happening in this country? Were the media so venomous about Trump that they were willing to destroy someone who wanted to help the country, regardless of politics?

It wasn't enough for me to point out over and over what I thought should be obvious—namely that I was asked to help precisely because I was in health policy, *not* epidemiology. To determine the best path forward in a health crisis with broad impacts and a wide array of possible responses, it should go without saying that government leaders must consult experts who could weigh the impact of the policies themselves. That's the role of policy experts like myself with a broader scope of expertise than that of epidemiologists or immunologists. And that's exactly why I was called to the White House. There were zero health policy scholars on the Task Force; no one with a medical background who also considered the impacts of the policies was advising the White House. And not once before my arrival did the harmful impact of the Task Force's draconian efforts to stop the virus ever get mentioned, let alone undergo detailed discussion, by any of the other medical scientists in the room.

The media properly should have been calling out the Trump administration for months over the lack of health policy experts on the Task Force. In the end, the most egregious failure of the Task Force was its complete and utter disregard for the harmful impact of its recommended policies. This was outright immoral, an inexplicable betrayal of their most fundamental duty. I have no doubt it will go down as one of the greatest public health failures in history.

Yet now, regardless of my position and expertise, I was to be discredited. Why? Because I had the audacity to step forward and help the country alongside a president whom the media despised. That meant I had to be delegitimized, undermined, even destroyed. After all, it could not be the case, *it must not be allowed to be true*, that this president was listening to legitimate experts, academicians of the highest level, scientists with national and international reputations. Absolutely nothing would be permitted to change their settled narrative that Trump "wasn't listening to the science."

Totally disregarding my seventeen years in health policy and full-time position in a public policy institute, the media did their best to pigeonhole me as a radiologist and breathlessly denounced me as "not an epidemiologist." Many times, I honestly wondered, who in their right mind would want health policy to be designed solely by someone as narrowly focused as an epidemiologist or a virologist or any basic scientist for that matter. I am still incredulous about that inane criticism, which I also heard repeated by former colleagues in academic medicine who rushed to discredit me because I had disregarded their advice to refuse to help the Trump administration.

The absurdity peaked when I heard what surely wins the prize for dumbest comment of the year about me from the press. In response to hearing my clinical opinion that we expected the president to recover from COVID and come back to work soon, Chris Wallace of Fox News blurted out to his Fox colleague, "He's not an epidemiologist!" As if the opinion of an epidemiologist on a clinical medical question would be more credible than a doctor with decades of experience consulting on thousands of patients with infectious diseases and other illnesses in the US and throughout the world. Wallace further exhorted his viewers: "Follow the scientists! Listen to people like Anthony Fauci. Listen to people like Deborah Birx!" People whose entire careers had been confined to bureaucratic agencies would be the ones to look to for clinical perspective, I guess.

Eventually, the bizarre "epidemiology" claim became simply comical. It's still a source of laughter in my family, who often start a joke by saying, "Well, I may not be an epidemiologist, but ..." In the end, it was like living in a Kafka novel, though with far more dangerous consequences. Major news journalists were so blinded by their political hatred, so willfully ignorant, perhaps so frightened themselves, that they could not process simple common sense. These people were the filters and purveyors of important information to the public. Hence, their ignorance generated even more fear in an extraordinarily fragile nation.

I still wonder how much lasting psychological damage was caused by the American media, especially to our younger generation. Adding to the lunacy, as my Stanford and Harvard epidemiology colleagues frequently reminded me, cackling through their laughter, they didn't even realize that Dr. Fauci was not an epidemiologist either—perhaps the one thing he and I had in common.

Meanwhile I was also taking fire from my colleagues back at Stanford. In September 2020, soon after I had been introduced publicly as an advisor to the president, a group of Stanford medical school professors issued and actively publicized a letter that advanced several false claims about my policy views. Claiming they were "calling attention to the falsehoods and misrepresentations of science recently fostered by Dr. Scott Atlas," they organized and disseminated their statement by Stanford's internal listserve email, and it was posted on a School of Medicine website—violating Stanford University policies while giving the false impression of an official institutional opinion. They were quickly forced to pull the posting down.

The Stanford Provost reprimanded them by writing, "You can use your University title and professional affiliations, however, you must make it clear that the views and opinions expressed are your personal views and do not reflect the official policy or position of Stanford…. In the last week, we saw an inappropriate use of our official Academic Council email list. A letter from some medical school faculty was written and signed, consistent with the freedom of faculty to voice their opinions. However, the letter was distributed to all members of the Academic Council using a University email list and that was not consistent with policy. That will not happen again."

Responding to their shockingly inappropriate letter, Dr. Joel Zinberg in a September 2020 piece in *National Review* called

"Cancel Culture Comes to Medicine" noted what was really happening. "Atlas has been singled out for professional erasure by 98 of his former Stanford medical, epidemiological, and health-policy colleagues because he had the temerity to join President Trump's coronavirus task force and advocate rational measures for safely reopening the economy." He also reprimanded Stanford by stating the obvious: "The academy is supposed to encourage and tolerate vigorous debate, not end it with mob condemnation. Experts can and do disagree in good faith over the next steps to be taken to handle Covid-19. Disagreement in good faith ought to be accompanied by full and open discussion, but that is not what the Stanford letter is trying to achieve."

Victor Davis Hanson, a distinguished scholar of history at Stanford and Hoover Institution, also called out "the unscientific attack on the science of Dr. Scott Atlas." He posed a question no one honestly needed to contemplate. "So why—other than politics—is there now a concerted media attack on Dr. Scott Atlas, an adviser to the Trump administration on COVID-19 policy?"

CHAPTER 8
Early Conflicts with the Task Force

Much had transpired in the White House Coronavirus Task Force in the six months before I began participating. Since the final days of February 2020, the Task Force had been led by the vice president when he took over from Secretary of HHS Alex Azar. Throughout the spring and into the summer, Drs. Birx and Fauci represented the Task Force, whether in the Oval Office or to the public in the media. Birx and Fauci stood alongside the president during headline-dominating debacles in the Brady Press Room about hydroxychloroquine, drinking disinfectant, ingesting bleach, and using UV light to cure the virus. They were there for a full six months as the sole medical input into the Task Force, generating the entire advisory output to states. Virtually all states implemented what Birx and Fauci recommended, rolling lockdowns. Their Task Force also had the logistical problems with testing and personal protective equipment (PPE) availability. They had fallen short, especially early on when testing would have been extremely impactful. And for months, they sent out mixed messages to the public, emphasizing uncertainty, highlighting what we didn't know rather than what we did, and inexplicably ignoring the massive body of acquired evidence and the compendium of knowledge about immunology, including related coronaviruses.

Before my first Task Force meeting in mid-August 2020, I had already been engaging in a back-and-forth with a friend in the White House for a few weeks. It was clear to him that the Task Force doctors were fixated on a single-minded view that all cases of COVID must be stopped or millions of Americans would die. In addition to the reck-lessness of such a narrow view, the cases and deaths had not stopped. The clearly identified high-risk people, including nursing home pa-tients who already lived in a controlled environment, kept dying from COVID. That ongoing tally of cases and deaths, presented 24/7 on the news, incited even more fear and led to meek acceptance that un-precedented, draconian shutdowns must be put in place.

Fear was the dominant mood throughout the country. No mat-ter what the president said about the need to reopen, the states were nearly all following the lockdown advice of Fauci and Birx with a handful of exceptions, like South Dakota, Florida, and a couple of others. Even after the president tweeted out contrary messages in April about "liberating" Michigan and Virginia, those states were kept under strict lockdowns, ultimately remaining so for the rest of the year.

For me, the different messages coming out of the administra-tion were puzzling. Wasn't the president supposed to be in charge of national policy? Of course, each state determined its own on-the-ground policies. Even Redfield told the press in August that the CDC was merely an agency issuing guidelines, not rules. Mean-while, the president had already been on record that he wanted to both protect the vulnerable *and* reopen schools and the economy.

Contrary to the stated policy of the president, though, the Task Force members were continually pushing their own advice to the public. The president advocated opening K-12 schools; Birx-Fau-ci-Redfield kept warning that schools should be closed because "we don't know for sure" about the risk to children. He stressed protect-ing the high-risk population while opening businesses and allowing healthy Americans to work; they wanted widespread testing and confinement of healthy people, with closures of business and sig-nificant restrictions on movement. Even on explicit mandates, they expressed their own views. The president had clearly stated his pol-icy on masks—he recommended them when you could not socially distance, as did the NIH, the WHO, and others; Birx, Fauci, and Redfield repeatedly pushed universal masks, even mandates, for ev-eryone, in interviews and to governors.

I often wondered why they wouldn't simply tell the president to his face they disagreed with him and at least have the integrity to say that if he wanted other policies, they would resign. Instead, they chose to stay and put forth mixed messages to the public. To me, this was extremely harmful. Presenting internal discord undermined public confidence in the management of the crisis, adding to public fear in an already politicized environment.

This schizophrenic messaging from the White House, I believe, represented one of the president's most significant errors of judgment. The way I saw it, the problem was the president's blind faith in those closest to him. He relied too much on his most trusted political advisors. I recognized that their intentions were to help him win the 2020 election; that was their job. Kushner, tired of my attempts to show him the data that refuted the lockdown strategies, eventually told me, "I am agnostic about the pandemic." But by focusing on the perception of voters instead of the data, the administration had elevated a couple of government public health bureaucrats to effectively be in charge of public policy. No matter what the president himself said, the vice president and the political team—almost everyone, really—feared Fauci and Birx, who held extremely high public approval. That was a de facto authorization, allowing them to formulate and then communicate what the public would hear as the administration's policy recommendations.

That autonomy was not just realized by Fauci and Birx; it was incentivized by the adulation they received in the media as they kept articulating opinions contrary to the president. As a result, a parallel messaging stream from the administration itself continually contradicted the president's own statements on the pandemic—including his correct sense that continuing societal lockdowns was severely harmful.

There were serious consequences from this pattern of contradictory information. It exacerbated the confusion in the public and increased the fear that the leadership was off-track. The voters' perception of Fauci and Birx handcuffed the messaging from the administration—except from the president himself, who continued to emphasize reopening with targeted protection of the vulnerable in all of his own remarks. Meanwhile, Birx, Fauci, and the vice president's Task Force were essentially on their own, presenting an entirely different message to the country.

That should never have happened. That was the job the president was elected for—to lead national policy, to make the decisions, especially in a crisis. And the more Fauci and Birx disagreed with the president's ideas, the more they were elevated by the heavily anti-Trump media and served as justification for the draconian edicts of governors and local health officials. Even to this day, that deference to Fauci and Birx, out of a desire to win the election, still paralyzes much of the American populace with fear. There will be long, lasting damage from the anti-science recommendations they promulgated.

Still, others more trusted by the president who should have known better were adding to the problem, whispering in his ear to echo the Fauci-Birx mandates, restrictions, and mass testing, regardless of the harms of the accompanying lockdowns. To me, the most surprising was Scott Gottlieb, former head of the FDA. No one could have thought his motivation was political. Gottlieb had already served in his role at the FDA, by instituting the president's policies of reducing bureaucracy and facilitating competition to reduce drug prices. I also knew him from past interactions on health policy. Indeed, I had thought highly enough of him to personally recommend him to be head of the FDA when the Trump transition team came to me searching for candidates. I do not think his views were clouded by being a board member of Pfizer, one of the key vaccine companies poised to benefit from special agreements with Operation Warp Speed. Because he was advocating the accepted fear-mongering narrative, though, no one ever shrieked, "But he's not an epidemiologist!"

By late July, the mostly silent dissenters inside the administration were even more convinced that the recommendations coming out of the Task Force were wholly misguided. Temporarily flattening the curve to avoid hospital overcrowding? That had become a distant memory. The goalposts had long since shifted to something very different. Now, the imperative seemed to be stopping all cases, period, even eliminating positive tests in people with zero symptoms and very little risk of any serious illness. Not only was this impossible, it was also irrational. This highly contagious respiratory virus was already widely prevalent, having infected tens of millions of Americans by estimates of the CDC and others. The overwhelming majority of infected people were asymptomatic or only mildly so. And experts on pandemic preparation in the past had never advised societal lockdowns—the severe harms were easy to anticipate and long viewed as unacceptable.

I later discovered that several others in the administration, including some in Task Force meetings and a few at the COVID Huddles, were similarly skeptical about the pronouncements of the Birx-Fauci-Redfield troika. Right from the start, staffers and officials working in various agencies and departments would call out my name as I walked back and forth to the West Wing or inside EEOB, expressing thanks and expressing relief that I had arrived. Some were seated at the table in those meetings, while others sat in the periphery as staff or representing federal agencies (HHS, CMS, OMB, CEA, and so forth). The problem was that none of these dissenters had medical backgrounds. Therefore, they were reluctant to voice concerns, knowing they could not possibly carry the day. They had also witnessed the unpleasant reactions from Birx whenever she had been challenged.

Although I was asked to come to Washington specifically to advise the president, Kushner insisted it was also important for me to participate on the Task Force. I had been working behind the scenes in the White House since the end of July, advising the president and working on policy initiatives. I immediately replied that it was not a good idea. Kushner was well aware, at least insofar as the president's own thinking was concerned, that the administration policy was to reopen schools and society. I believe he naively thought "the doctors" could be convinced by the data and my perspective.

I, however, was convinced that it would only result in personal conflicts without any impact on policy. Wasn't it clear that Birx and Fauci were all-in on their lockdowns and what I would call "unfocused protection" by this point? Their strange shift from flattening the curve to maintaining that we must stop all cases of COVID-19, at all costs, was firmly set in stone. It did not matter that their policy was failing to save lives while simultaneously destroying lower-income families. Dr. Fauci himself called it simply "inconvenient," seemingly without any self-awareness that he spoke as a member of an elite class. Surely, if Birx and Fauci ignored all the data that was contrary to their policy, including months of experience from all over the world, why would they suddenly rethink everything? Why listen to me, an outsider?

In the middle of my initial Task Force meeting in mid-August, I realized that my assumptions were correct—nothing good would come of my being on the Task Force.

* * * * *

For months before coming to Washington, I reviewed the data every morning and multiple times per day. By late spring, I had developed dozens of contacts with other researchers, many of whom filled my inbox with more accurate analyses of trends every day. In addition, unbeknownst to most people, a large number of private individuals throughout the country had been painstakingly analyzing source data and then recalculating and posting the more accurate dates of cases, hospitalizations, and deaths. In my mind, these are among the silent heroes of the pandemic. Many had backgrounds in data, statistics, or math; others were simply concerned citizens, critical thinkers with the common sense to question the status quo. These valuable relationships continued while I was in the White House, providing me with data that was entirely unknown to Birx and the others on the Task Force. That stream of information was critical, because all predictions and policies were geared to the trend lines, including the claims about the impact of mandates and lockdowns. If the trends were not reflecting the situation accurately, then all bets were off regarding the assessment of those policies.

From early on, I knew that sources such as "worldometer" and most government websites were neither sufficient nor accurate. It was already common knowledge that data dumps and dates of recordings were rife with errors. For instance, a sensationalistic headline blaring the record number of deaths on one day in Florida represented a report of deaths from several different days over several weeks that had been "dumped" into the records that day. I was surprised to see Dr. Birx, the main disseminator of "the data," routinely distribute curves from worldometer and state dashboards at Task Force and COVID Huddle meetings without ever noting their inaccuracy. This was the tip of the iceberg, but I didn't know it at the time.

Just before I arrived in Washington, I received a July 20 email from the White House asking for my comment on what Birx was claiming about Arizona. She wrote, "We modeled masks, no large gatherings, closed bars and reduced indoor dining which Arizona did 3 weeks ago. They should have over 5198 cases daily and climbing and they have less than 2000/day and declining so it's not just Europe—we now have evidence in the US and we left retail open, people working it's just the bars and large indoor gatherings. But if we have masks in public everywhere including indoors then you really only have to close bars and limit indoor dining. This is working, it's a translation of science into real life practice."

This write-up illustrated a fundamental flaw in models of the pandemic, one certainly not unique to Dr. Birx. Like many others, she thought proof of impact was that a smaller number of cases occurred than was predicted by her model—a model with its own built-in assumptions of how many cases would be found without certain interventions. It was bad enough that the example was accompanied by a printout of what looked like worldometer trends. This conclusion was inherently nonscientific—modeling that something might occur, and then because it did not occur with a given intervention, concluding that the intervention was effective. That was not proof of anything at all; it was circular reasoning. Why couldn't the explanation be that the model's prediction was wrong? Indeed, modelers had concocted a scenario in which cases would keep spreading as if everyone was equally susceptible, without regard for increasing immunity or seasonal effects—all known to have occurred in every respiratory virus pandemic over the past 130 years. These models were grossly incorrect, as later proven by numerous publications showing the lack of impact of lockdowns.

Even if that circular reasoning was disregarded, to claim cause and effect from a correlation was frighteningly simplistic. Scientists learn early on in their training that "correlation is not causation." Websites listing spurious correlations were widely known, because even very strong statistical correlations between wholly unrelated trends could be easily found. During my time in Washington, my colleagues at Stanford and elsewhere routinely commiserated with me about this lack of critical thinking about the pandemic.

The first item on the Task Force agenda was nearly always an update by Birx on the data and on her travels. There was no question that she worked very hard; indeed, every morning by 6:00, Dr. Birx was already sending out her emails of compiled numbers. While she regularly related a few experiences from her visits, she proudly reminded everyone that she "was all about the data." What was not outwardly acknowledged was that her data was mainly a compilation of automatically generated tabulations of cases, hospitalizations, and deaths, as well as some percentages and trend plots. The set of data she distributed always included arbitrary categorizations of the cases, test positivity, or other factors in specified ranges that were assigned certain colors. Convenient to look at, those categories were not of sound scientific basis; nothing formed the limits of the ranges other than arbitrary cutoffs. Yet these categories automatically garnered significance and drove meaningful policy decisions at the state and local levels.

The charts were also distributed by Dr. Birx in the regularly held COVID Huddles, generally run by Kushner. These gatherings were mainly geared to coordinating the group of nonmedical people outside the Task Force in preparation for messaging and public events. It was only related to the Task Force by the presence of Birx and then later by me, too.

I soon came to understand that Birx's summaries of each state's trends had a major impact on their implemented policies. It was not simply that internal White House email recipients or Task Force attendees received her charts. She was the "official" representation of the Task Force outside Washington. She worked very hard at disseminating advice to each state, spending a huge amount of time flying around the country, speaking with governors, meeting with the regional and state authorities, visiting college campuses, and appearing on regional media. Dr. Birx herself, to my knowledge, composed documents for each state, which were assumed to represent advice from the Task Force. Those sheets were at times also distributed to the Task Force and COVID Huddles, especially if an upcoming event would be held in those states. At the top, whatever trends she compiled were put forth. At the bottom was a set of specific statements—advice on personal behavior, mandates, restrictions on businesses and schools. That advice was authored by Dr. Birx, one of her responsibilities.

For starters, the lengthy data summaries, tabulations, charts, and plots were essentially recapitulations of data sourced from the very states that received the summaries. As I had written in an email on my very first weekend in Washington, "The key thing that B should be doing is interacting with states to instruct them on how to refine their data (e.g., separating hospitalized patients due to COVID symptoms from hospitalized patients who happen to have a positive test)." But no. These were mainly just reorganized and reformatted numbers—which were then sent right back to the states that had originally supplied them on their various websites.

I didn't need to point out the other absurdity of her recommendations—one that was brought to my attention, very directly and in no uncertain terms, by several governors. More than once, I listened to outraged calls from these governors. On one hand, governors were frustrated by her repeated idiotic reminders to wash hands or use social distancing. "Scott, does she really think we need to hear what we already know, what everyone is already doing??" More than one governor told me they refused to have her visit their state. "She is going on TV, telling everyone that we should have mask mandates, pushing her pseudo-science, hectoring college students," one told me, subsequently telling the VP's scheduler that "under no circumstances will she be allowed to visit the college campuses in my state."

Yet, true to form, key political advisors of the president and the VP were walking on eggshells, afraid of alienating Dr. Birx. They told me directly that their main concern was the upcoming election. When I asked how to deal with angry governors, the VP's chief of staff, Marc Short, said in his office, "Scott, I absolutely agree with you, you are right about focusing on protecting the elderly, the lockdowns are destructive, we must open schools. I am living that myself."

VP Pence himself also assured me that the data and policies I expressed were correct; he had requested from me, and personally read, summaries of studies and documents on schools, risks to children, testing, and other issues. Given that the VP was in charge of the Task Force, shouldn't the bottom-line advice emanating from it comport with the policies of the administration? But he would never speak with Dr. Birx at all. In fact, Short, clearly representing the VP's interests above all else, would do the opposite, telephoning others in the West Wing, imploring friends of mine to tell me to avoid alienating Dr. Birx. I assumed his concern was the obvious— the election was approaching.

It did not matter one bit that he was convinced the science supported my policy advice, nor did it matter that my advice matched the preferences of the president. Marc Short and Mark Meadows both emphasized to me that regardless of any policy disagreements between myself and Dr. Birx or Dr. Fauci, even in the face of their overt distortions of my views, I must not say a word. "We cannot rock the boat!" To which I would reply, "The boat is frigging capsized!"

I soon understood why many others invited to the Task Force didn't even bother to attend its meetings after a while. Yes, many on the Task Force were highly competent and productive, like those at FEMA and elsewhere who were working on logistics, PPE manufacturing and distribution, prioritization of equipment and testing to where it was needed, tracking of economic indicators by the CEA, OMB, and the Department of Labor, as well as many other areas. I enjoyed working productively with several Task Force members on important steps to bolster the protection of high-risk populations, including Seema Verma of CMS, and at times others. Moreover, the vaccine work under Operation Warp Speed especially was proceeding rapidly, although there were some delays that were not easy to explain if not for politics. No doubt, though, the president and many others understood that listening to the public health discussion in the meetings were often less than an optimal use of time.

What bothered me the most was the absence of discussion about the research, the unsophisticated thinking about the data, the lack of attention to detail about the studies. Just one important example was the discussion of risk factors for death from COVID. In addition to the most important factor—age—everyone also knew about "underlying co-morbidities," added risk from other conditions. And by then, most observers further understood that obesity, diabetes, cardiovascular disease, and some others were on that list of risk factors. However, more detailed epidemiologic analyses, including Williamson's publication in July 2020, had shown that high blood pressure alone was not necessarily a significant risk factor for death from COVID. That would have been extremely important to the tens of millions of Americans with well-controlled hypertension. Instead, a false impression that all "underlying conditions" were equally significant as risk factors was left as fact. After arriving in the White House, I was surprised that no medical Task Force members expressed any detailed knowledge about the research on risk factors beyond broad strokes reported in the media. Even after I brought it up several times at COVID meetings, with the printed-out publications in hand, it was never commented on—other than the glare from those insecure about having their lack of knowledge exposed. To me, that was not the expected level of legitimate scientists, let alone those supposed to be advising the president of the United States and the nation.

Even allowing for a non-expert level of knowledge, the Task Force doctors somehow ignored the evidence indicating the very low risk from this infection for the overwhelming majority of people. Birx even emphasized at the Task Force that this infection was extremely dangerous exactly because it was so commonly asymptomatic or so mild that it went unnoticed—*as if it would be less dangerous if it were more deadly*. There was no articulation of what we knew, what the scientific studies and the world's evidence had shown. On the contrary, Fauci repeatedly emphasized in his occasional Task Force comments, as he did in his frequent media interviews, what we did not know with certainty, just as a layman without any medical perspective would do. For instance, the issue of risk to children, or spread from children to adults, was always, "Well, we don't know for sure," despite repeated studies from all over the world elucidating that we did know. That pattern of highlighting uncertainties while minimizing decades of fundamental immunology and virology was alarmist and contrary to the expected behavior of a public health leader. It created massive fear inside and outside the White House, and it drove on-the-ground lockdowns and mandates. That failure in turn diverted the focus to exceptions and rarities, like the multisystem inflammatory disorder seen in children or the incidental cardiac MRI finding in asymptomatic young patients.

Because there was almost no citation of current science by the three main medical voices on the Task Force, I made sure to bring stacks of published studies to every meeting. In fact, I was the only person who ever brought scientific articles. My briefcase was filled with reprints from scientific journals, explanations of the pitfalls of testing techniques, manuscripts and essays from epidemiologists and medical researchers, and charts compiled for comparison of issues relevant to the Task Force. For what I anticipated would be a data-filled discussion about opening schools and the risk to children, I brought approximately fifteen different studies and a summary sheet of the research. For what I hoped would be a discussion about testing guidance, I brought and distributed articles and other documents about the role and pitfalls of PCR testing and concerns about cycle thresholds. Even though I handed out a number of these published studies to everyone at the table, no one ever mentioned them in the Situation Room. My guess was that no one in the Fauci-Redfield-Birx troika ever opened them.

* * * * *

My first foray into the Task Force was mid-August. My West Wing friends empathized, because they already knew what awaited. The Task Force had been meeting for more than six months by then, and my colleagues were well familiar with the history that preceded me.

Regardless, my friend John Rader, a key source of positive energy, smiled broadly and wished me good luck. Derek Lyons, the staff secretary, chuckled knowingly behind his desk. I walked down the short hall, briefcase stuffed with papers clutched under my arm, toward the Situation Room.

I said hello to several who were already in the room and spotted my placard at my assigned seat. After a couple of moments, Vice President Pence and his staff entered. We all stood. He introduced me to the group with a warm welcome; he was always very kind to me. I consciously planned to say very little. I was new, so I thought I would just observe for now.

Birx began, as was the rule, with her overview of numbers—trends in infections, hospitalizations, and deaths. She recited her favorite statistic, "test positivity"—the percentage of tests that came back positive. That always struck a chord with me, because that percentage was also a reflection of the total number of tests. Sure, it indicated the number of positives, but the percentage would be totally different depending on how many tests were performed and who was tested. Testing was not at all being done in a controlled, statistically valid way, using representative population-based sampling, like surveillance testing. The percent positive, therefore, had questionable value, whether in comparing different states or even in the same state, since nothing was standardized or constant.

She then stressed the need for social distancing, handwashing, and masks. I wondered why this still needed to be emphasized to this group, as if it was somehow a new idea to the Task Force. They had been meeting for more than eight months, and the nation had been hearing this virtually 24/7 in all media outlets. Her mantra of "keeping cases down" with mass testing of asymptomatic people and quarantining of all those testing positive was then repeated, and repeated again.

Then a jarring claim was made. Dr. Birx began talking about "the Sunbelt"—in particular, Arizona—and said, "We brought down cases there." Echoing statements in the July 20 email that I had been sent weeks earlier, she claimed that Arizona proved that certain closures worked, including closing bars and reducing indoor dining at restaurants, along with mask mandates. Why? Because her estimates of cases that *would have* occurred, by her model, never did. Instead of continuing to escalate, cases started declining. It apparently didn't even register to her that these curves were characteristic in every other state and virtually every other country. Instead, this must prove that the masks and other imposed restrictions had prevented them.

I stayed silent. I had analyzed the Arizona data in far greater detail, but I didn't want to begin with a huge disagreement. Birx then pushed for imposing those same restrictions everywhere, specifically bar closures, restricted restaurant hours of operation, and mask mandates. It struck me that everyone, including the VP, said nothing at all or subtly nodded their heads, particularly Redfield and Fauci.

The acceptance of such blatantly flawed conclusions by the people formulating policy at the highest levels was deeply disheartening. Didn't she see that the cases declined in a similar pattern in places with very different policies? Why did everyone ignore that their prescribed lockdowns were not protecting the elderly, who were still dying? No one voiced any concern at all about the health harms to individuals, families, and employees of such closures and restrictions.

Moreover, the Birx-Fauci-Redfield recommendations to maintain business closures, severely restrict personal activities, and issue mask mandates were adding to the public's fear, because they directly contradicted the stated policy of the administration, thereby creating more uncertainty and fueling the sensationalistic media. In my way of thinking, if they had sound science to back up their contrary policy and dispute his ideas, those points should absolutely be raised with the president himself. Shouldn't they make their case directly to the leader of the administration? And if the president disagreed, they should resign—because no one with any professional integrity could stay on in that event.

But that was not their course of action. Their comfort with contradicting the president's stated policies now was especially striking, given that months before I arrived he had made far more controversial suggestions, including drinking disinfectant and self-medicating with hydroxychloroquine. Yet they were apparently afraid to speak up then, when it was clearly needed, as public health officials on national television.

Meanwhile Birx went on. Without anyone challenging her or even asking any questions, she reiterated the need for even more restrictions, specific limits on the operation of restaurants and bars, and maintaining school closures. Pence looked around, saw the nodding heads implying agreement, and said, "I guess everyone agrees."

I strongly disagreed, but I remained reluctant to speak. I was there for the first time. I wanted to avoid arguing, and it would be impossible to pose this as a minor point of disagreement. Thankfully in retrospect, Pence noticed the look on my face and said, "Scott, I asked you here because I want to hear your opinions. Say what you're thinking." He used his favorite phrase, used many times in the Situation Room—albeit to no discernable effect—"I believe iron sharpens iron!"

Of course, the VP was right. No matter how uncomfortable this would undoubtedly be, I had to speak up. So I began with the two words I would say in almost all of these meetings—words that would become a running joke with my friends in the West Wing: "I disagree." I continued to explain, very calmly, all the while knowing this would not go over well. "I disagree that 'we brought cases down.' That was the typical curve of the virus. It came down for other reasons—almost everywhere in the world had demonstrated a characteristic curve. I think the drop was due to acquired immunity from enough people getting the infection in the local population in that region, and some was due to seasonal factors."

I maintained my gaze on the VP as I continued. He was listening intently.

I then explained a fundamental flaw in many trends being highlighted in the media, known to everyone doing hands-on analysis of the data—but apparently unknown to the doctors in the room. Cases were already coming down in Arizona on day one of the governor's mask mandate. Birx's dates were wrong, so her trends weren't accurate. I had gone through this in painstaking detail days earlier with one of the many outside analysts who were working with me. The cases in Arizona had already peaked and begun to decline before the governor's statewide universal mask request could possibly have had an effect, i.e., the same day of the governor's announcement.

More fundamentally, even after more than six months of looking at the numbers every day, Dr. Birx apparently didn't realize that reported dates on most government agency dashboards and in the media at the time, like the COVID Tracking Project, were misstating actual event dates. Instead, many websites reported events by the dates of recording. That generated two important errors. First, the death totals recorded on any given day really represented deaths spread out over weeks, some dating back even months. Second, the peaks were falsely shifted. That shift of the peak was usually at least two weeks—all because of relying on recorded date instead of the date of the actual death. This represented one of the most misleading inaccuracies in the reporting. Headlines blazed about spikes in cases or record numbers of daily deaths, yet the spikes were often artifacts of reporting patterns. Since trends were being used to define almost all policies, those trends absolutely must be accurate. But they were incorrect.

I chose to avoid explaining her second serious mistake, which derived from a naive reliance on correlation—i.e., believing that a chosen correlation proved causation. This kind of unsophisticated reasoning was frequently demonstrated by the Task Force medical troika as they voiced similarly invalid conclusions about masks and lockdowns in subsequent meetings, conclusions that were so obviously unsound that they were questioned even by the nonscientists around the room.

I then talked about New York City, where Birx had also claimed that cases were declining due to government-issued mask mandates. I said, "I disagree that cases came down in NYC due to masks." I hadn't brought my chart with me, but it would have been almost cruel to point out the fact that the mask mandate for New York was on April 15, yet the cases had peaked weeks earlier and were already in steep decline. I instead pointed out there were almost no cases now, for several months, even after thousands had joined arm-in-arm in the streets, shouting in megaphones, even sharing them, in large crowds with zero distancing. In fact, there were so many infections that serology studies showed a fairly high prevalence of antibodies. I mentioned some of that antibody data—but no one in the room had bothered to consider it, though it was publicly available. One study had been published in *Annals of Epidemiology* showing that in New York City, about 23 percent of residents already had antibodies after the spring wave. It was well known that antibodies generate protection; that was basic immunology, not new science to be discovered. Moreover, studies from La Jolla, Karolinska, and elsewhere had shown that approximately double the percentage of people showing antibodies were also protected by T-cells, including people without antibodies or even known exposure to the virus. I explained that if 20 percent had antibodies, then about 40 percent more had T-cells; so that implied that about 60 percent of a population had protection.

I also went into a very simple explanation of the concept of herd immunity, since dozens of people were listening to this meeting. Most in the Situation Room had no medical knowledge, and the overflow room and many on the video and audio connection had none, either. I explained that if a large enough percentage of people had antibodies, they block the pathway of spread, thereby preventing the unprotected from getting infected. This was high school biology, not esoteric knowledge.

Not once did I advocate allowing infections to spread—not in that meeting nor in any other meeting, and never to the president. This was only an explanation of a biological phenomenon, a well-known one at that. Despite what was later reported, there was nothing remotely controversial in what I actually said that day.

I mentioned that I had even reassured my own family six months earlier that New York City would end up being safer before anywhere else. My guess was that we likely would not see a massive spike in the next several weeks, due to getting closer to herd immunity. I repeated the very basic point that Sunetra Gupta had explained on May 21, that "much of the driving force (of cases coming down) was due to the build-up of immunity." In fact the hardest-hit communities in NYC now had a very high prevalence of antibodies, significantly higher than more affluent neighborhoods, so they would be more protected from the next wave, assuming one occurred. I had brought the numbers on antibody testing in NYC, by age and income group, but I knew the data from memory. Again, Birx said nothing about the antibody data; neither did Fauci or Redfield.

Dr. Birx, seated diagonally across the table, was glaring at me. I asked her, very directly, why she thought NYC had no cases after their first massive wave of hospitalizations and deaths—in the face of huge crowds protesting in the streets, with all that entailed. I asked, "Do you think masks brought the cases down?" Birx was visibly angry. She insisted I was wrong. She raised her voice and angrily snapped, leaning forward, "Yes! And because of the lockdowns!!"

I went on to briefly make the case that we should not lock down everyone, since that was enormously harmful. Instead, we needed to do a better job protecting the high risk, with far more diligence. Their indirect protection strategy was not working—it was in place nearly everywhere in the country, yet the elderly kept dying, and meanwhile society was being destroyed. Schools were closed, even though kids had such low risk. Their strategy was being implemented, and it was not just failing to save the elderly. The Birx-Fauci lockdowns were killing people, destroying families and children from skipped medical care, generating massive psychological harms, heartbreaking drug and child abuse, and quantifiable lives lost from unemployment. How did I know this? I had done the research myself in collaboration with scholars from three other academic institutions. I had analyzed the data in detail on the harms of the lock-down, and I had written a paper on it earlier. The others on the Task Force clearly had not.

Everyone was basically frozen; tension filled the room. No one offered any study or data to refute the severe harms of the lockdown or anything else I said. I felt a pit in my stomach, seeing how angry Birx was, particularly since this was my introduction to the group. But I reminded myself that this was why I was asked to participate. Their biggest problem was not simply that they were not epidemiologists, an irony unrecognized by the press. The problem was that I was the only *health care policy* scholar in the room. I was the only one there with a medical background who also considered the enormous health impacts of the Birx-Fauci policy *itself*.

Once the meeting adjourned, I left the Situation Room without lingering. I naturally assumed no one else agreed with me. After all, no one had said a word; no one either agreed or disagreed with me other than the interruptions and protestations of Dr. Birx. As I marched down the hall I felt a little dejected but also angry. These were "America's best doctors"? These were the people advising the president of the United States and counseling the governors drafting edicts throughout the nation? These were the people entrusted with the public's confidence, placed on a pedestal as experts, to advise us in the biggest health crisis in a century? I never saw them act like scientists, digging into the numbers to verify the very trends that formed the basis of their reactive policy pronouncements. They did not act like researchers, using critical thinking to dissect the published science or differentiate a correlation from a cause. They certainly did not show a physician's clinical perspective. With their single-minded focus, they did not even act like public health experts.

Later that day, I spoke with a few others who had been in the room, people in high level positions, including advisors from HHS, economists from OMB, and Marc Short, the chief of staff for the VP himself. They individually expressed almost the exact same message: "Scott, thank God you're here; I've suspected this for months."

The truth is that I was the only doctor in the room who ever spoke about the health harms of the lockdowns, a fact that weighed heavily on me every day during my time in Washington. Perhaps I was the only one receiving hundreds of emails per day from people all over the world—parents, pastors, students, school board members, active and retired teachers, even senior researchers at NIH—relating their personal tragedies. People pleaded with me, exhorted me, even begged me in emotional terms to keep speaking out about the suicides, depression, lost businesses, crushed families, the desperation of their elderly parents, all because of the lockdowns. While Birx, Fauci, and Redfield focused solely on stopping cases at all costs, in media interviews and in their advice to governors, pushing their brain-numbing message of "wash your hands, stay away from others, wear your masks," I was the only doctor representing the White House who also explained to the public, providing data in written pieces, in interviews, and through the president's remarks, that the lockdowns were destroying people. Now I more fully understood the importance of my being there, exactly why I was brought into the White House.

* * * * *

Several days later, before the start of a Task Force meeting, Dr. Fauci handed me his personalized NIH note card with his handwritten cell phone and email. He asked me to call him later; I made the call, sitting alone in Rader's office, since it was right down the corridor from the Navy Mess. It was all very pleasant and collegial. Fauci explained that he wanted to talk, to see "if we had common ground," and asked me a series of questions.

He first asked, "Do you believe in any of these mitigation measures at all?" He wanted my thoughts about social distancing, handwashing, group gatherings. "Of course I am for those!" I responded, stunned at such a strange question. I had interviewed and written dozens of times, specifically agreeing with mitigation measures, and especially protecting the higher-risk people with even more measures. My concern was that the lockdowns were ineffective and were also severely harmful—literally killing people. That mattered, didn't it? I knew right away that Fauci was way off base in his assessment. He evidently assumed from my caricature in liberal media that I was some of kind of ignorant right-wing science denier.

We then spoke about kids and schools, and he asked what I thought "about the risk to children." I went through a fairly thorough discussion of the international literature to date on the remarkably low risk to children for serious illness or death. Off the top of my head, I listed studies from more than a half-dozen countries that showed the lower rate of spread from children, including contact tracing data. I mentioned the Swiss study showing that school was the source of only 0.3 percent of infections. I described data verifying the absence of unusually high risk to teachers. I was doing almost all of the talking. Fauci listened. He offered no other studies, no other data, and nothing in dispute, other than commenting, "Well, what if we aren't totally sure?" I was taken aback, because this was not the sort of thought process I anticipated in a data-driven scientist or public health expert.

He also brought up testing. I gave him my thoughts on the consequences of testing and confining people who were not symptomatic, the data on asymptomatic spread, and what I had learned from my discussions with John Ioannidis and Jay Bhattacharya about the limits of contact tracing at this point in a pandemic. Fauci never expressed a single word of disagreement. Zero contrary data or publications were cited to indicate any divergent opinion. In fact, there was no back and forth on any of these topics. There was never anything I perceived as a scientific interchange. It was all one way, from me to him. Our conversation ended very amicably, though.

Afterward, while having my snack in Rader's office, I happened to glance at the news reports. I was astonished. It turned out that Fauci had alerted the media beforehand that he was going to talk with me that day. I wondered, "What kind of person would give a heads-up that he was going to speak with me?"

I shook my head, reminding myself that I simply do not fit in with these people. I finished my cheese and crackers, then went back to looking at data about Texas and Florida.

* * * * *

Soon it was time for another Task Force meeting. The VP wanted to talk about schools and the risks to children, among other things. But first, as always, Dr. Birx provided her update—numbers, trends, and some anecdotes from the road. As always, Dr. Birx included her color-coded tabulations using numbers she had compiled in a stack of charts and tables already distributed to everyone seated. As always, she emphasized "test positivity"—the fraction of tests that were positive. That was the magic number, in her mind. This was also emphasized in the COVID Huddles, and no one among the communications team knew enough to question its utility.

By this time, I had pointed out to whoever would listen that the percent positivity was unreliable, because it was highly dependent on who was tested and on the amount of testing. The problem with relying on statistics like that one was well understood by data analysts outside the administration. For instance, if we mainly tested sicker people in that state, then test positivity would likely be higher than in a different state. Or if we only tested fifty people per week in a state, and ten were positive, that's 20 percent—very high—and could vary enormously from a week with 10 percent, even if the difference was only five positive tests. That would have very different significance compared to a similar percentage change in another state with a far more robust testing program of, say, ten thousand people per week. Separately, and not uncommonly, many states posted "data dumps" for their test results—lumping results together on Mondays, for instance, even though those tests were performed on several preceding days. Not to mention that PCR tests were conducted with very different sensitivities from lab to lab and state to state. Even beyond those problems, it was not uncommon that some labs only reported positive results. These innumerable distortions had no impact on discussions in the White House, however.

Dr. Birx reported, as she always did, that she had been reinforcing the message about standard mitigation measures on her travels. But it always struck me as very odd, given that by now all states were already using those measures. I wondered if she hadn't heard what I had already heard an earful of from a couple of governors who called me to say they were frustrated and angry. "Does she really think we still need to hear to wash our hands and socially distance?" After listening to their complaints, I would talk to them about their hospital bed situation, whether they had a shortage of PPE materials, and how to limit spread to nursing homes by testing the staff far more frequently, every day, if they had a high infection level in the community. The disgruntled governors would also share their impressions of the damage the lockdowns were causing in their states. It was my impression that most governors sincerely wanted assistance on designing their states' response; instead, they were receiving basic admonitions and unscientific rules, as though they were children.

Then Birx mentioned the topic of masks. My previous remarks on this subject were still in memory, I was sure. Everyone had already heard me mention that several states, countries, and cities had cases rise and fall regardless of mask mandates. This time, it was Redfield's turn to chime in. He had surprisingly prepared something in advance and pulled out a single sheet of paper, representing data from one state, and announced, "I have proof that masks work." What struck me was the irony of the situation. These people had pontificated about "the science" of masks for months. Redfield had even coauthored a July opinion paper, before I came to Washington, stating that masks were not only proven to decrease cases, it was "a civic duty" to wear them. Yet he only now found it necessary to show evidence to justify the policy—based on case trends in a single state? I looked around, with that "am I the only one seeing this?" bewilderment. I was apparently the first person in the Task Force who had actually challenged the assertion, which is shocking in itself.

Dr. Redfield proudly waved his chart around, holding it up for everyone in the room. He pointed at the chart it displayed and said, "Look, here is when the mask mandate came into effect; and see, this curve shows cases came down." I said nothing. This was not "science" in any sense of the word—it was embarrassingly simple-minded. But I did not want to be the only one pointing out the unscientific acceptance of a cause-and-effect relationship merely because it fit his desired correlation. He made no attempt to compare this data to another state, let alone to any controlled experiment with and without masks.

Fortunately for me, someone else in the room couldn't resist. Marc Short, the VP's chief of staff, politely raised his hand. "Excuse me, Dr. Redfield. Why couldn't that just be the normal decline of cases that we see everywhere, over time?" Redfield had no intelligible response. After a few awkward mumblings, we moved on to the next agenda item.

* * * * *

Near the start of the next Task Force meeting, Dr. Fauci excitedly exclaimed, "Scott, this may interest you," from across the table. "There is a report about myocarditis in these patients." This was truly remarkable, in one sense. It was the only time I can recall during my entire four months in the White House that Anthony Fauci spoke up about a research study.

Fauci began by explaining that an MRI study showed myocarditis in people after COVID. From his vague description of it, I assumed that he got his information from a summary, rather than the entire research report. I had read this study. I knew the methodology and the results in detail. I had already discussed it with cardiologists and infectious disease physicians who took care of patients. And I had previously authored scientific papers on MRI abnormalities in people without symptoms—the essence of this small report—so I had a thorough understanding of its implications.

I politely listened as Dr. Fauci spoke about the study. He quickly jumped to what he often did—the alarmist interpretation of "how dangerous this virus is." He then moved to other things "we don't know," speculating about potential problems from this virus. He then garbled out something that was almost unrecognizable. He had grossly mispronounced a medical term.

I leaned forward, struck by what I heard. I interrupted. "What did you just say?" He stopped immediately, frozen. No reply.

I repeated my question. "What did you just say? What are you trying to pronounce?" Fauci just looked at me. The room was silent. Then I said, "Are you trying to say *encephalomyelitis*?"

This was an uncommon inflammation of the brain or spinal cord that could occur after a viral infection. Uncommon, but well known to doctors with clinical medical expertise. I had published and taught about encephalomyelitis for decades.

I needed to clarify the meaning of the findings, since I was concerned that Fauci would issue his usual alarmist proclamations on cable news. I spoke for ten straight minutes, explaining the study design and the data. None of the twenty-six patients had clinical myocarditis. I further explained that this is not how medicine is practiced. Doctors do not actively seek an imaging finding in asymptomatic people, especially using an exquisitely sensitive test like contrast-enhanced MRI, and then conclude that these asymptomatic patients have a clinically significant illness. In fact, we often see "incidental findings" of doubtful significance in people scanned for other reasons, and I gave examples. I also pointed out that even using far less sensitive techniques (EKG and blood tests), even the flu is associated with clinical myocarditis—a frequency that undoubtedly would be far higher if MRI was performed in everyone testing positive for influenza. This small report of four entirely asymptomatic individuals with an MRI finding after COVID was absolutely not a cause for alarming the public.

I stopped. No one said a word. Birx, Fauci, Redfield, Giroir—none of them said anything, because they had nothing to contribute. We went on to the next agenda item, and the meeting eventually wrapped up. Within thirty minutes, I received calls from three others who had sat through that debacle. All of them thanked me, relieved that someone actually with medical perspective had spoken before misguided public statements were made.

*   *   *   *   *

At a subsequent meeting, now a full nine months into the pandemic, there was still a remarkable lack of certainty about the very policies they had been recommending on a daily basis. Even though they constantly invoked "the science" in their interviews, they grasped at straws to prove the value of their recommendations. Once again, assertions about masks were brought up, because the spread had not been stopped. It must not matter to them, I kept thinking, that most people were already wearing masks and that mask mandates had been put in place in dozens of states and in most major cities. I had demonstrated in a series of charts from cities, states, municipalities, and countries that cases surged right through several weeks or months of mask mandates. That included Hawaii, LA County, Miami-Dade County, Alabama, several European countries, and numerous other locations. This was empirical data—not models, not hypothetical projections, not opinion. Nope, it simply *must* be that people were not wearing masks!

Again, I was the only one with data, including the May 2020 CDC review showing that masks had no impact on either transmission or infection by influenza, a similarly sized virus. I cited the Oxford University review of all mask studies. I also recited mobility data on how restrictions had objectively limited activities, and national and several regional surveys all showing that mask usage was high. The data did not matter, though. They simply ignored the evidence. Again, Dr. Birx interrupted, as she commonly did, and glared at me. "You should really get out there more; it's not true." To her, apparently, it was not "all about the data" anymore. It was now about anecdotes.

As we were perusing some other charts in the packet from Dr. Birx, Dr. Fauci spoke up. Just like Redfield had done a few meetings prior, Fauci declared, "I have proof that masks work." Again I wondered, "Wasn't that 'the science' six months ago, when they all advocated universal masks?" Fauci continued, without any charts or data, remarking on a comparison of two neighboring states, one with and the other without a mask mandate. The state with a mandate had a slightly earlier decline in cases per day.

I was not going to bother arguing at this point; it seemed futile. But others by now had become emboldened to express their doubts. It took a nonscientist to point out the lack of critical think-ing. CMS Director Seema Verma interrupted. "Tony, you know that is not a valid comparison; those states have so many differences, in population, in urban versus rural counties, in demographics, in weather. There is no way to claim that difference is due to masks." Fauci had no reply.

No further comment was made on the matter. And again, the doctors in the Task Force showed no study about mask efficacy or any other of their policies, and they never once mentioned the harms of the lockdowns that I witnessed. Their sole focus was stop-ping cases, even when their policies were already implemented and were failing to do so.

* * * * *

The usual discussion began, with more updates from Birx on cas-es, hospitalizations, and deaths. Certain regions and some specif-ic states were highlighted as problematic areas. More restrictions, with an emphasis on restaurants, were called for. It was also very important, she again emphasized, to close bars at a specific time. I think she proposed 11:00 p.m., although at some point that changed to 8:00 p.m. As usual, I wondered where "the science" came from when it came to determining the precise hours when bars should be closed. I found myself pointing out that the data about bars showed something different. I cited contact tracing studies from Switzerland showing that a grand total of 1.6 percent of cases began in bars and restaurants. Regardless of their claims, however, no one in the Task Force cited data about bars spreading more cases after specific hours.

Once again, their assertions were wrong and their policies ca-pricious and arbitrary. The absence of spread from bars was later corroborated in December 2020 in New York City by a contact trac-ing study, showing that restaurants and bars accounted for less than 2 percent of new COVID cases. Likewise, in November 2020, LA County data showed that restaurants were linked to less than 4 per-cent of coronavirus outbreaks in *all* nonresidential settings.

As often happened, Fauci spoke up to support Dr. Birx's concerns, saying people need to be warned even more strongly about the dangers of the virus spreading, about wearing masks and distancing. He claimed Americans didn't think the virus was serious, and that was the reason cases spread. I was honestly surprised. I thought people were already panic-stricken. Normal life had virtually ceased to exist, even eliminating serious medical care or last visits with dying family. Meanwhile the media were on-message 24/7, instructing the public about masks and social distancing; there were signs and announcements demanding masks and diagrams about distancing everywhere; healthy young people were outside riding bicycles or driving their cars alone, wearing masks. Indeed, surveys showed that most adults perceived grossly exaggerated risks, particularly but not only younger people; and yes, a high percentage were obeying the edicts, distancing and wearing masks, according to virtually every published survey.

I challenged him to clarify his point, because I couldn't believe my ears. "So you think people aren't frightened enough?" He said, "Yes, they need to be more afraid." To me, this was another moment of Kafkaesque absurdity. I replied, "I totally disagree. People are paralyzed with fear. Fear is one of the main problems at this point." Inside, I was also shocked at his thought process, as such an influential face of the pandemic. Instilling fear in the public is absolutely counter to what a leader in public health should do. To me, it is frankly immoral, although I kept that to myself.

* * * * *

Several days later, I took the elevator down to the lobby in the Trump Hotel, where I was now living, to have a quick breakfast. On the wall behind the bar, adjacent to the dining tables, hung four massive television screens, one of which was always tuned to CNN and another to Fox News. Headlines were filling the screens, starting with the *Washington Post*, breathlessly quoting "several anonymous sources" said to be in the room who claimed I was "advising that we should let the virus spread" or "advocating a herd immunity strategy." Of course, I had never said anything like that, not even remotely advocating that the infection be allowed to spread. To the contrary, my public record was filled with specific advice to use mitigation measures and calls to increase those protections for the vulnerable population.

I was shocked and amazed by this public attack from my colleagues. But at the same time I knew that it was not just an attempt to demonize me, to falsely portray me as reckless, but an attempt to hurt the president politically. I am trying to have everyone consider all health harms of the policies and the virus, the only one trying to save lives from all causes—but I am being portrayed as endangering people?? Americans, already off the rails about the pandemic, fragile and filled with fear, were now going to think that his hand-picked advisor actually wanted the infection to run wild through the population. "My God," I thought. "Truth did not matter one bit to these people. They had no shame when it came to achieving their goal; they lied and distorted the facts without any concern whatsoever about its effects."

A few days later, it happened that Fauci and I were entering under the West Wing awning at the same time. I turned to him in the foyer and demanded to know, "Did you tell the press that I was advocating a herd immunity strategy? Did you say that?" The tone in my voice made it obvious that I was angry. He immediately replied, "No, that wasn't me. I never said that!" I found that hard to believe, but admittedly, there were dozens of people listening to the earlier Task Force discussion.

I also suspected that Dr. Birx was one of the people who fed that to the media. She had sent email just days before to the Task Force and COVID Huddle participants, warning that "2.2M deaths" would occur in the next few months "if everyone was to become infected." The most revealing part of her email, separate from the mistake of relying on a widely disparaged model, was her innuendo "these types of comments are not helpful," as if someone (me, I realized) had advocated some sort of "let it rip" scenario to achieve herd immunity.

Fauci seemed to be the obvious candidate. As the preferred source for almost every media outlet, I had seen him almost every day on the ubiquitous four-in-one White House television monitors, often several times per day. He had asked me straight out if I had no belief in mitigation measures in our recent conversation, implying that was what I believed, though I immediately corrected him. He had also personally alerted the press before any conversation even occurred.

Absolutely incensed, I continued. "I hope you're not the one. You *know* that's not what I believe. I'm disgusted. I've never worked with liars like this before, people who would make stuff up and spread it to the press." Without another word, I turned away and headed toward the Situation Room.

Regardless of whether it was Fauci, Birx, or both, the "anonymous sources" episode had enlightened me. My theory was that with them, it was not political; it was all about their egos. I guessed that they were threatened when challenged on scientific grounds and maybe also annoyed at being sidelined from public visibility at the president's side. To me, their remedy was simple: destroy me in the media. This was apparently standard practice in Washington, but it was foreign to what I had experienced in my academic career. There, to win an argument you made sure to read more, to know more, to analyze the facts. It was not about delegitimizing the other person. If you walked into a meeting, you had better be prepared, because plenty of other smart people were in that room to challenge you.

Regardless, I reminded myself of what was really important. The Fauci-Birx policies were implemented in almost every state, and those policies were destroying the country, literally killing people. When I entered a Task Force meeting, I would now consider these people in an entirely different light.

CHAPTER 9
Debating "the Science" about Schools

By the time I arrived in Washington at the beginning of August, it was inconceivable to me that in-person schools had been closed in the United States. It had already been proven months earlier that children were at extremely low risk of serious illness from COVID, and they had almost zero risk of death. That was indisputable scientific fact, based on an extensive body of published evidence from the US, including the CDC, as well as from all over the world—Finland, France, Germany, Spain, Sweden, Switzerland, Canada, the Netherlands, Iceland, the UK, Australia, Ireland, and many more countries.

Most European nations had opened their schools, because those countries did not deny the data about children. CDC had acknowledged that "[COVID] deaths of children are less than in each of the last five flu seasons" and "for children (0–17 years), cumulative COVID-19 hospitalization rates are lower than cumulative influenza hospitalization rates during recent influenza seasons." As exemplified by the conclusion of a study of the pediatric hospitals in North America in *JAMA Pediatrics*: "Our data indicate that children are at far greater risk of critical illness from influenza than from COVID-19."

The month prior to my arrival, there had been efforts to push for school reopening by the president and the administration. News coverage had highlighted disagreements between the president and the CDC guidelines at the time, guidelines that included significant behavioral restrictions on young children, like distancing and masking. According to CBS news reports at the time, CDC Director Redfield put that into appropriate context, explaining that the guidelines were just that, guidelines and not requirements. That critical perspective about CDC guidance has unfortunately been missing from virtually every subsequent discussion about the management of the pandemic.

By the end of July, even the CDC finally acknowledged what had been known throughout the world for months—that "COVID-19 poses relatively low risks to school-aged children." I pointed out this logical disconnect about schools in *The Hill* at the end of July 2020: "The logical implications of these belated declarations are striking: If steps need to be taken to protect children from COVID-19, then those same steps are required each and every year that the influenza season arrives, a disease that kills more children, that causes hospitalization of more children and that is frequently transmitted from children to the same high-risk teachers and family members who then die." Of course, we would never close schools annually for seasonal flu.

All who bothered to look also knew that it was extraordinarily harmful to children to close in-person schools. By summer, evidence had accumulated that long-distance learning was a failure. Learning was in free-fall. In Boston, only half of students were showing up for online instruction on any given day; 20 percent had not even logged on. Virginia's state school superintendent commented, "This situation is going to be like what is often called the summer slide [in student achievement], but on steroids." Teachers reported in a May 2020 survey by EdWeek Research Center that students were spending only half as much time—three hours per day—learning. A Center on Reinventing Public Education survey documented that only one in three districts even expected teachers to use their teaching materials, with rural and small-town districts far less likely than urban and suburban districts. Fewer than half of all districts even communicated the expectation that teachers would take attendance or check in with students regularly.

Even worse, school closures were widely recognized to be more destructive to working class and poorer children. All the academic losses were recognized to be more severe for children in less affluent families. Districts with the most affluent students were twice as likely to require at least some teachers to provide live, real-time instruction. The director of the Center on Reinventing Public Education at the University of Washington Bothell noted that kids in urban districts may have lost 30 percent in reading proficiency and 50 percent in math. She warned the House Education and Labor Committee in testimony that without a major improvement, students could descend into "academic death spirals." Not to mention that jobs of working-class and less-affluent families, especially single-parent homes, would be paralyzed if children were not able to attend schools.

Additional serious harms from in-person school closures were all predictable and began to pile up. It was common sense that kids would not possibly learn normal social skills, like working in groups, resolving conflicts, or simply making new friends. And the children who depended on schools for nutritional needs or for discovering the need for eyeglasses or hearing aids were now ignored.

Data was also showing increasing psychological harms from isolation, with skyrocketing calls to suicide hotlines, doubling or tripling of symptoms of depression and anxiety, social withdrawal, and suicidal ideation. Doctor visits for self-inflicted harm in teenagers were later documented to have been soaring, more than tripling where lockdowns were most severe. And precipitous drops of reported child abuse cases were documented—hundreds of thousands during the spring of 2020 school closures alone—since schools are the number one agency where such abuse is noted.

These almost unspeakable increases in domestic abuse were known to correlate with unemployment and the attendant stresses, all of which were far worse for lower-income families. This was an unmitigated disaster and was noted as such by the American Psychological Association, the World Health Organization, the CDC, and throughout the nation's—and the world's—expert journals and public health agencies.

The icing on the cake, given the enormous social harm of closing schools, was that children were not likely to spread significantly to adults. This was not the flu, where kids were often the source of spread to adults. This data was clear from the science reported throughout the world's literature. Studies from Finland, Sweden, the Netherlands, Switzerland, France, the UK, and elsewhere confirmed the fact that children were almost always infected from adults, not the other way around; that few cases originated in schools; that teachers did not have higher infection rates than those in any other occupation; and that school "outbreaks" were typically just positive tests without any symptoms or only mild illnesses.

Even if children did transmit it to adults, however, that was not a reason to keep schools closed. On top of that, teachers in the US were typically young, not high-risk individuals. Yet this hypothetical danger, flying in the face of all data, was clung to by school-closure advocates as *the key reason* to close schools. Indeed, America was unique among all our peer nations in being willing to sacrifice its children out of fear for adults; most European countries had reopened their schools.

I had already expressed frustration in multiple interviews that anyone who called for in-person schools to be closed was not prioritizing children. In a series of interviews, I repeatedly raised an obvious question, one that was never answered: Wasn't educating children an essential social function? After all, other essential businesses were operating. By that time, I had received dozens, if not hundreds, of pleas from parents all over the country, imploring me to fight to open schools. Even several teachers and school board members contacted me, shocked at how schools were closed, uncertain what to do. Several were instituting lawsuits to force schools to open; a number contacted me to help with expert testimony.

Many top epidemiologists and infectious disease scientists, including Harvard's Martin Kulldorff and Katherine Yih, Oxford's Sunetra Gupta, and Stanford's Jay Bhattacharya, were also speaking out on the imperative to open schools. Closing schools was indefensible on both moral and scientific grounds. Yet, inexplicably, America's schools remained closed.

During my first few days in the White House, prior to my first attendance at a Task Force meeting or a COVID Huddle, we began planning a White House event to highlight "School Reopening." I quickly took on the task of drafting initial details for a structured event including outside medical experts, school administrators, and parents, all in attendance with the president, vice president, and Secretary of Education Betsy DeVos. And it certainly helped my case with the White House communications team that on August 3, the president had tweeted, with three exclamation marks, "OPEN THE SCHOOLS!!!" This was an opportunity for the White House to lead the call for what I felt should be one of our top national priorities, opening in-person schools. And given the compelling nature of the evidence, I hoped it would turn the tide.

I first outlined that the basis of President Trump's policy rested on three fundamental truths:

1) Children have extremely low risk for any serious illness, hospitalization, or death from COVID-19—less than seasonal influenza.

2) Keeping schools closed inflicts massive harms on children.

3) Educating America's children is a top national priority, far beyond an essential business.

I intentionally did not include the established fact that children did not significantly spread the illness to adults. That was not a prerequisite to opening schools in-person but a point of rebuttal for those opposed to doing so, especially teachers' unions. Harmfully, the media helped incite this baseless fear as they focused on the "risk to teachers" and the potential for children to spread the disease to their parents.

In the document that was later edited by several people and released by the White House, I drafted comprehensive policy recommendations for all schools, along with explicit support for parents to choose distance learning as their preference. That included guidelines to protect high-risk students and teachers; student age-based policy differences; and suggestions for group activities and school nurses. I carefully crafted detailed guidance for topics such as "Handwashing, Social Distancing, and Masks" and "Monitoring Symptoms and Signs." These policy suggestions were circulated to dozens of people in all the health agencies for edits and comments. In that and all subsequent drafts, diligent mitigation efforts, including handwashing, social distancing, and mask wearing "if unable to socially distance," were recommended for all teachers, staff, and high-risk students. Careful monitoring to ensure that symptomatic kids stayed home was highlighted. Healthy students were urged to be aware of hygiene; mask availability, handwashing stations, and open ventilation were also stressed.

The guidelines matched the guidance listed by Toronto's renowned Hospital for Sick Kids in their Recommendations for School Reopening of June 2020. In their document, they stated that "non-medical and medical face masks are not required or recommended for children returning to school" and provided eight bullet points supporting that recommendation. They explained that "facial expression is an important part of communication which children should not be deprived of." They also advised "strict physical distancing should not be emphasized to children in the school setting as it is not practical and could cause significant psychological harm. Close interaction, such as playing and socializing, is central to child development and should not be discouraged."

On August 12, 2020, President Trump unveiled the White House guidelines on reopening schools at a press briefing. Reuters covered the announcement, and their first sentence revealed the obsession with masks that had overtaken the entire pandemic narrative: "U.S. President Donald Trump on Wednesday released eight recommendations for reopening U.S. schools amid the coronavirus pandemic, including that masks be used when social distancing is not possible."

The event was held that same day, timed to follow up on the vice president's roundtable on school reopening three weeks earlier with South Carolina Governor McMaster. The president, vice president, Secretary DeVos, and several invited parents, teachers, and outside experts spoke on the urgent need to get children back to school. Kellyanne Conway moderated smoothly, as always, with a series of questions to highlight the benefits to open and the harms of preventing kids from being in school. The president interacted directly with several parents in the room, some with special needs kids, who gave compelling reasons why their children needed in-person learning and other important at-school activities.

One education policy expert, Paul Peterson, director of the Program on Education Policy and Governance at Harvard University, outlined the harms when children were prevented from attending school. A mother and neonatologist, Dr. Melanie Piasecki, echoed a key point we also stressed—that parents should still have the choice to opt for distance learning, if that suited their family's needs.

Toward the end, the president, as he often did, turned to me for spontaneous comments. I took the opportunity to restate the key points behind the policy of opening in-person schools. "We know that the risk of the disease is extremely low for children, even less than that of seasonal flu. We know that the harms of locking out the children from school are enormous. And we also know, as we all would agree, that educating America's children is right at the top of the list for our nation's priorities." The president concluded by advocating for society opening up broadly, and he briefly mentioned opening college football.

Everyone thought the meeting was a great success—with the exception of the press, who did their best to denigrate the idea of opening schools, to instill fear into the public by emphasizing this was "even though cases were high in the community," and to totally ignore what had been clear from the scientific data. At the time, though, I thought to myself, "Progress!" But while this overwhelming body of evidence was consistent and widely published, it would be another full year until the case for reopening schools was admitted to be compelling by the mainstream media.

*　*　*　*　*

The vice president's office had placed K-12 schools on the Task Force agenda. And for good reason. America was off the rails and uniquely so about schools. While most of our peer nations in Europe had opened schools for in-person attendance, the US had tragically decided the opposite. Based on fear, and directly contrary to the evidence, shuttering in-person schools during the late spring was the policy implemented by almost all school districts. Virtually the entire world's science overwhelmingly said to open in-person K-12 schools.

Even after the excellent July 23, 2020, CDC publication acknowledging the importance of opening in-person schools and the harms of school closures, there remained an insistence inside the Task Force, particularly by Birx but echoed by Redfield and Fauci, that we must double-down on school testing, quarantining, and significant mitigation efforts, even by young children—even knowing that they interfered with learning and normal socialization. For anyone who fully thought through such a policy, the testing and quarantining of asymptomatic children would inevitably lead to one thing, school closures.

When the VP came to K-12 school policy as the next agenda item, he called on me to speak. He knew that I felt strongly about this issue. It was not just because the scientific case was so clearcut. It was another surreal misapplication of common sense, one that totally defied logic. Schools were indeed unique—uniquely *low* risk. The biggest difference between a school and elsewhere was that schools were *lower*-risk environments, *less* dangerous than the surrounding community. We knew children had an incredibly low risk from this virus. The idea that children represented a serious danger to adults was also directly counter to all the world's data. One of the largest studies in the world on coronavirus in schools, carried out in one hundred institutions in the UK, confirmed that "there is very little evidence that the virus is transmitted" in schools. Children had even been called "brakes" on the spread of the infection by researchers in Germany. Yet, somehow, in the minds of this team of public health leaders, we needed to focus even more on schools—increase testing, increase PPE, and increase restrictions. Meanwhile these wrongheaded views were uncritically amplified by American media.

In anticipation, I had brought more than a dozen studies to the meeting, published articles from scientific journals and government websites, but I didn't pull them out.

First, I explained (with numbers) that children did not have significant risk of serious illness or death from this virus. I cited statistics from New York City, California, and elsewhere showing almost zero risk of death. I noted the data from Sweden—zero deaths, despite schools not closing and not requiring masks. I further explained that the harms to children of closing in-person schooling were widely documented, not just in the CDC publication. They were extensively illustrated, dramatic and irrefutable, and included poor learning, higher drop-out rates, depression and anxiety from social isolation, and massive numbers of unreported child abuse cases. Most of these serious problems were far worse for kids in lower-income families.

The icing on the cake was the evidence that almost all coronavirus transmission to children comes from adults, *not* the other way around. That was not a predicate for opening schools, given the massive harms to kids if they were closed. But that evidence was already shown by contact tracing and other studies in Iceland, Canada, France, the Netherlands, Germany, Sweden, Finland, Ireland, Japan, Switzerland, and elsewhere. Opened schools and childcare centers did not show significant dangers to children, adults, or teachers. I didn't bother critiquing the two studies—Korea's and Israel's—purporting to show the contrary. Those were already shown to have been incorrect. For instance, upon reanalysis of a recent Korea study, those authors had issued an addendum to correct their first conclusion that had claimed children spread as frequently as adults. That study generated false, alarming headlines in the *New York Times*, but a corrected analysis showed only a single case of a child passing on the disease to another household member—

and that was to another child. They found zero instances of a child passing the infection to an adult. Likewise, the media had done great damage by sensationalizing the Israeli experience, claiming erroneously that school openings were the source of subsequent community infection outbreaks. But that assertion was false, as I demonstrated by analyzing their social mobility tracking, wherein all sectors of society in virtually the entire country had opened with extensive social mingling for the weeks prior to schools opening.

As I finished, there was silence. No one offered any contrary data. No one spoke of scientific studies. No one even mentioned the discredited Korea study. Zero comments from Dr. Birx. Nothing from Dr. Fauci. And as always, not a single mention by Birx or Fauci about the serious harms of school closures. In my mind, this was bizarre. Why was I the only one in the room with detailed knowledge of the literature? Why was I the only one considering the data on such an important topic with a critical eye? Were the others simply accepting bottom lines and conclusions, without any analytical evaluation? Weren't they supposed to be expert medical scientists, too? I waited.

In response, Birx told me that my opinion was out of the mainstream: "There is a bell curve of epidemiologists, and you are at the fringe." (Hadn't she heard that I was not an epidemiologist?) Meanwhile she insisted that all experts agreed with her. I shook my head, thinking of some of the world-class epidemiologists who agreed with me—John Ioannidis and Jay Bhattacharya of Stanford, Martin Kulldorff of Harvard, Carl Heneghan and Sunetra Gupta of Oxford—and wondered if she or Fauci had ever read a single publication by them.

The vice president thanked me and looked across the table, turning the floor over to Dr. Redfield as director of the CDC, the agency that issued guidelines on school openings. "What are your thoughts, Bob? What do you think about the risk to kids, about opening schools?" I looked to my left; Redfield leaned back and stroked his chin. "Let's just say, the jury is still out." End of discussion.

I was disgusted at Redfield's apparent lack of knowledge, shocked at his ignoring the scientific studies that had been published from around the world. I looked around the room, wondering if anyone else understood the glaring incompetence on display. Clearly, Pence needed more input.

*   *   *   *   *

By this time, I had alerted several of my colleagues outside Washington about the incredible assertions that totally contradicted or frankly denied science that had been bandied about at the Task Force. They empathized but strongly encouraged me to stick with it. One renowned epidemiologist wrote, "Ugh! I now know what you're dealing with." Then he offered to come to DC and personally meet with the others on the Task Force: "Birx and Fauci are not epidemiologists. I do not know if they are open to and interested in learning more about disease outbreaks, or even if that would help. If you think they are and it would, and if there is any way I can contribute, let me know."

That was perfect timing. Fauci had contacted me again. We spoke on the telephone. Fauci offered a proposal. He said it might be a good idea for "the doctors on the Task Force" to meet "to see if we have common ground." I envisioned the three-on-one encounter. Given that I had already attended a few Task Force meetings, I had a hard time being optimistic about how that might go. I also had experience with these "colleagues." In all likelihood, my statements would be distorted and then funneled to their favorites in the press. More distortions, more defamation, more character assassination would ensue.

How did I know what would follow? It had already happened. After the widespread repetition of distortions and lies about my words on "herd immunity" put forth by the *Washington Post*, the *New York Times*, and CNN, I was receiving vile, hate-filled emails, many that included death threats. The FBI and White House security had already been alerted and were monitoring the situation. And from those irresponsible hit pieces, I had experienced unhinged

Washingtonians screaming their profanities into my face in public; "Trump lies, people die, fuck you!!" one screamed, leaning into me as I ate Indian food with friends outside in an upscale neighborhood, and "Fuck you, herd immunity!!" as I walked with someone in a quiet neighborhood. Not to mention the secondary impact, a truly depressing indictment of the despicable side of American culture—the Twitter lunatics who were on the prowl with their vicious, irrational attacks, foaming at the mouth while bizarrely failing to see that the Birx-Fauci lockdowns were in place nearly everywhere and those policies were failing to stop people from dying, while destroying families and children. I was in no mood to trust these three doctors to keep such a meeting internal.

But I had my own idea, a way to have something positive emerge. I replied enthusiastically, "Sure, absolutely we should meet!" I said I thought it was a great idea. And I proposed to him that I would have a couple of top epidemiologists also attend, so we could jointly go over the data in detail, have a thorough discussion on the science. These would be medical scientists who were actually publishing research on the pandemic, I noted. In fact, I had already mentioned the idea to two of them, I told Fauci, and they were ready to fly to Washington. After all, what scientist wouldn't want to discuss the data with some of our nation's top academic epidemiologists during a national crisis?

Fauci weakly replied, noncommittal, but clearly he was caught off-guard. He quickly ended the call. In the end, he dropped the whole idea and never brought it up again.

* * * * *

In addition to K-12 schools, of course, the Task Force was equally concerned with colleges and universities. It was critical to address this issue quickly, because colleges were starting to reopen. A basic tenet in this country is that higher education is a gateway to opportunity, integral to the economic development and future leadership of our society. It was clear that if colleges were not opened, not only would we fail to educate our next generation of leaders, but also we would seriously harm our younger generation's entry into the workforce. Moreover, like other school closures, all the data showed the negative impact of closing colleges was worse on lower-income students and minorities.

Ironically, the policy of searching for asymptomatic cases among college students was endangering high-risk Americans. In fact, I had just held a lengthy telephone discussion with an Ivy League university provost the previous weekend. He proudly described his detailed COVID protocol, filled with required serial testing, quarantines of asymptomatic students, strict limits on all social interactions, and an absolute refusal to allow students to use any university resource or enroll at all unless they cooperated fully with his plan.

I asked if he understood the risk to students was extremely low, even if they were infected. I reminded him about the pathway his testing regime necessarily led to. That is, if we extensively test healthy, low-risk students and then find asymptomatic cases, we would react by quarantining healthy students. Since they would have interacted with others, we would find even more positive tests, again among perfectly healthy, asymptomatic people with very low risk. Inevitably, that would lead to closing campuses. The next step, of course, would be to send the students home—the exact opposite of what we wanted to do if we were interested in protecting public health. By sending kids home, they would be removed from the safer, extremely low-risk college environment and sent out to a higher-risk environment, their homes and communities with older, more vulnerable individuals. The provost politely acknowledged these issues, but he proudly restated how "successful" his policy had been, because they had not experienced major "outbreaks" on his campus—indeed, he was pushing it to be the model for all Ivy League schools.

In advance of our meeting on colleges, Birx distributed her email update to the group, as well as to COVID Huddle participants. In it, she noted the "worrying signs across the USA from rising cases in college towns." I had been following the campus data very closely myself. A research professor who had been assisting me since before I arrived in Washington was regularly sending me updates. I had all the details on college student cases, hospitalizations, and deaths.

At the meeting, I recited the facts about the campus numbers. I explained that the sensationalistic phrase "school outbreaks" was itself misleading—these are typically cases detected only by testing, not clinically significant illnesses. Thousands of cases were reported from campuses across the country, yet almost none actually needed medical care. Of the first 11,000 "cases" as defined by positive tests, zero were hospitalized. Soon over 25,000 cases—positive tests in mostly asymptomatic students—had been registered. Yet with all those "cases," zero hospitalizations—no illnesses requiring significant medical care.

My view was that there was an alarming disconnect between the data on risk to college-age individuals and the policies being implemented. I pointed to the CDC statistics, that only 0.2 percent of the first 164,280 deaths catalogued by the CDC had been in those under twenty-five years old. For those eighteen to twenty-nine, that risk is 90 times less than for those sixty-five to seventy-four, and 630 times less than for those eighty-five and older. I noted that hospitalization rates for those eighteen to twenty-nine are very small compared to older age groups: one-eighth of those seventy-five to eighty-four, and one-thirteenth of those over eighty-five. And I spoke about the relevant demographics on campus: that 90 percent of full-time students in public colleges are under twenty-five, and 98 percent are under thirty-four; that few university faculty members were elderly, since two-thirds are under fifty-five years old, and only 13 percent are older than sixty-five. The risk to that age group was extremely low, and the campus was one of the lowest risk environments one could imagine.

Dr. Birx strongly disagreed about the significance of campus cases. She warned that once college students get cases, they spread the infection to the community. "Cases lead to hospitalizations, and hospitalizations lead to deaths." No one would claim that deaths did not arise from hospitalizations or that hospitalizations did not arise from cases. That is exactly why we must make sure policies, like massive testing, did not lead to the dangerous consequence of closing colleges, something that was already happening. Closing campuses pushed students from their low-risk environment back into the community, where high-risk people lived.

My second point, totally ignored by everyone else in the room, was that the policy of locking down younger adults to stop the entire population from acquiring a virus that had been shown to be spreading despite all efforts was severely harmful. That was a proven failure. Instead, I said, we should devote as many resources as possible to protect the high-risk people directly—targeted protection—and stop destroying the health and livelihoods of everyone else.

No one on the Task Force presented any data. No contrary evidence was mentioned. Warnings, broad statements, and assertions were uttered, but never any data or evidence.

Finally I offered my opinion as to a reasonable campus policy guidance: students should use the standard mitigation measures, and when they are sick, they must isolate and stay away from class. Instead of panicking about cases with either no or mild symptoms that will generally resolve, schools should implement mitigation measures to diligently protect high-risk students and faculty; maintain reasonable limits on indoor groups; hold large group activities outside; and treat the symptomatic patients when necessary. I also echoed the practical concern, as expressed by former Indiana governor Mitch Daniels, the president of Purdue University, in an interview I had seen. We should monitor closely to prevent hospital overcrowding, an unlikely occurrence.

The VP finally chimed in. Logic had won! He firmly agreed with the most important part of the advice from the Task Force to colleges—we needed to do everything we could to keep students on campus. Everyone around the table nodded. This was great news, I thought. Despite the inevitable closings that mass testing would lead to, it would really help if we could unify around the key message: don't close the schools.

The VP assigned me and Birx to draft a short policy statement to then circulate around, with the goal of sending a one-pager to colleges and universities. A small group of us—the VP, Dr. Birx,

Dr. Redfield, and me—would subsequently hold a nationwide conference call with leadership in higher education, including college presidents, provosts, and other key administrators, to reinforce the importance of keeping colleges open.

We held the call in early September, after the VP's office finalized the recommendations stressing the need to maintain open colleges and universities. Alongside both Dr. Birx and Dr. Redfield, I spoke to the thousands of higher education leaders, explicitly noting the need to follow all recommended CDC mitigation protocols. I stressed the importance of protecting high-risk students and faculty members. Most important of all, I said it was critical to keep the campuses open, because college and universities were low-risk, safe environments compared to communities and homes.

I also prepared an op-ed on opening colleges and universities. It was submitted in the standard protocol I experienced during my few months there. I wrote it and sent it to the Staff Secretary. That office sent it to dozens of people of their choice in the administration for edits, which took several days. Eventually it was sent out and published by the *New York Post*. It was a very solid, highly referenced, data-filled piece. And it was filled with the right reasons for opening, and opening safely, including the use of all CDC-recommended mitigation measures and extra precautions about protecting vulnerable people.

The president underscored the point at his later press briefing, to reassure parents and students as kids returned to campuses. He showed a chart documenting tens of thousands of college cases, explaining that while we call these positive tests "outbreaks," they almost never result in any hospitalizations, let alone deaths. Nevertheless, the media kept pushing sensationalistic headlines about "the new campus hot spots" and tallying up "outbreaks" as the number of cases increased. To report objectively and reassure the public, the media should have reported that there were no deaths and only two hospitalizations out of more than 48,000 positive tests. That was never noted, let alone emphasized.

* * * * *

At our next meeting, Dr. Birx was traveling, so she called in from the road. The vice president thanked her for her tireless work, as was his custom, and then handed it over to "Deb." "Thank you, Mr. Vice President, sir!" she began cheerfully over the speakerphone. After her usual overview of trends and color-codes, she focused on her visits to college campuses.

Birx was describing what she insisted was truly dangerous about the virus on college campuses: it was so mild, so benign, that the overwhelming majority of college-age students never even noticed that they had it. They either had no symptoms or, at worst, were temporarily under the weather. She seemed mortified at their ignorance. Remember, these campuses already understood that the students must remain in the low-risk campus environment rather than go back home. "They don't even know they're sick!" she exclaimed, repeatedly, and laughed at what she thought was so absurd about it.

I began to look around the room. Was anyone but me hearing this? She was claiming this was a total disaster, a terrible situation, for the very reason that no one became ill. I checked out Fauci, Redfield, others in the room. Most were nodding, smiling broadly, several were even laughing along—these students were so silly to think there wasn't a huge problem.

Birx declared, almost frantically, "We really need to start testing the toilet water from the dorms, the drainage from their sewer system! Otherwise, we will never find the cases! No one will know they had the infection!"

I was speechless. No one made a comment to indicate they had heard anything odd at all.

But then she took the conversation to a new level of absurdity. Birx noted what she called "an alarming trend"—the ratio of "hospitalizations per case" was rising. She listed several states with increasing "hospitalizations per 100,000 cases." All attention was focused on this new trend. Birx specified that the total number of hospitalizations was not higher, i.e., *there was no increase in hospitalizations at all*. That meant this was not a worsening of anything meaningful.

There was no increase in total deaths, either, she stated. Regardless, she reiterated her concern—the ratio was increasing, and her solution was to increase testing of nonhospitalized people.

A number of others chimed in, expressing their concern. The vice president, Fauci, Redfield, and Giroir all nodded affirmatively. Some muttered something to the effect that this was indeed a very serious issue. I kept thinking, "Wait—there is no increase in hospitalizations; there is no change for the worse in any way. More testing will not identify any new hospitalizations; it will only reduce a fraction by increasing the size of the denominator. There is no new trend, because the number of hospitalizations has not changed at all."

Birx then repeated her remedy. We must increase the testing. Again, the other doctors around the table concurred. Fauci nodded. Giroir and Redfield strongly affirmed this solution. The VP agreed, looked around the room, and gravely stated, "Yes, we absolutely need to increase the testing."

I finally jumped in. "Let me point out something here, if I may," I began. All eyes turned to me. "Does anyone here understand what's going on? Does anyone realize the logic here, the circular reasoning? Is your concern here about the perception of a fraction, that the ratio of 'hospitalizations per 100,000 cases' is higher? Cases are defined by the number of positive tests, as we all know. Dr. Birx just showed that the number of hospitalizations is not higher. *There are no increases in sick people.* There is nothing concerning here."

No one said a word. I continued.

"Do you all realize that the purpose of testing is not simply to reduce a ratio? You are proposing to increase testing for one reason—to increase the denominator in order to bring down the ratio of hospitalizations per case. But the point of testing is not about changing a ratio. *Your solution of doing more testing will achieve nothing other than to reduce that fraction—it will not change the number of people being hospitalized. We already have noted that there is no increase in sick people.* All patients coming to the hospital are already being tested. There will be no consequence of doing more testing other than to lower that ratio. Your sole point is on changing a ratio by increasing the denominator of a fraction, not on helping anyone. That will change nothing."

No one said a word. Birx, Fauci, and Redfield were silent. They offered no rebuttal nor any defense of what they had accepted beforehand. The VP looked around but said nothing. After a few moments without comment from anyone in the room, the VP went on to the next agenda item. As the meeting ended, the VP noted, "So we will make sure we increase the testing."

I left the meeting. By now, I surmised that these people were simply incapable of basic logic, as well as unarmed with sufficient knowledge to debate. Within the next half hour, two others who had been in the meeting came over to commiserate with me, shaking their heads in disbelief.

CHAPTER 10
The Talented Dr. Redfield

One day in mid-September, I was munching my daily cookie in Rader's cramped office while watching Dr. Robert Redfield, director of the CDC, testify to Congress. Just one week before, the country had witnessed Redfield's bizarre testimony about masks that included some of the most ignorant comments imaginable by anyone purporting to be a scientist, let alone a holder of one of the most influential public health posts in the nation. His claim that "if every one of us [wore a mask], this pandemic would be over in eight to 12 weeks" flew in the face of empirical evidence from several US cities and states, as well as countries all over the world in which widespread mask wearing failed to stop cases from increasing. In that same Congressional testimony, Redfield famously insisted that "this face mask is more guaranteed to protect me against COVID than when I take a COVID vaccine." That was demonstrably false, a historically ill-informed statement that not only contradicted science, but heinously endangered those at risk to die.

Redfield's words simultaneously undermined the confidence in the forthcoming, highly effective vaccine while falsely emboldening the elderly's risk tolerance from their masks. I remember two acclaimed scientist colleagues asking me that same day, "What the hell is Redfield talking about?"

Redfield was also quoted as stating that it would not be until "deep into 2021" that Americans could even get access to a vaccine. That directly contradicted the time lines generated from information we all had heard about the clinical trials, as well as the clearly written production and distribution arrangements with the pharmaceutical companies that I had seen with my own eyes. That Redfield statement, too, was ultimately proven wrong.

Ironically, within days, Redfield was overheard by a reporter on a flight saying, "Everything Scott Atlas says is false." Bringing the Task Force discord to the press served a politically useful narrative of undermining the administration, so the press ran with it. But politics was not Redfield's motivation. Redfield had been exposed in the Task Force meetings since I came aboard. No one had ever challenged his statements or showed scientific data in the discussions. I guess I was a threat to his personal credibility—a threat to his status and the other members of the medical troika. Since they couldn't argue on the data, they used their ace-in-the-hole, the media. At least he was consistent in his uncanny ability to be completely wrong.

The very next day after his testimony, I also had to respond to his gross errors in a TV interview. As head of the CDC, Redfield had a high level of credibility, so his statements undermining the vaccine and its time line were impactful on the US and indeed on the entire world. Coming from him, that sort of misinformation was extremely harmful—the public was already frazzled, and the vaccine was key to the hope of a return to normal life. Moreover, I knew the correct information directly from the HHS team and had stated it on the podium.

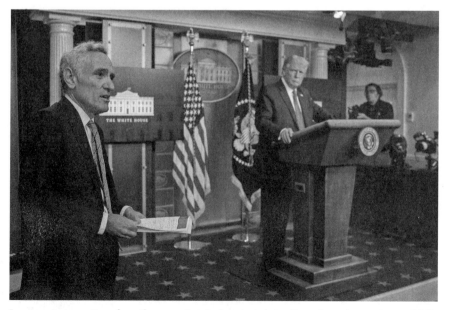

In answering questions from the press, I recited projected timelines about the vaccine availability and other operational details directly from White House documents, while President Trump watched from the podium. (*Credit: Official White House photographers*)

As I had specified, we could know if a vaccine was developed successfully in October or November; once that was known, the logistics had been set up so that first injections would be made before year's end.

On a Martha McCallum Fox News interview in follow-up, answering her direct question about his vaccine projection, I tried to soft-pedal a direct conflict. Regarding a vaccine not arising until late 2021, I answered, "No, because that's not the statement I was told by the people in HHS who are doing the vaccine deployment. I just got the information from them yesterday before the press conference. So, I'm not sure exactly what he meant or where he got his information. I'm not disagreeing with him; I don't know who told him that," I added. "All I can go by is what I was told." I did not want to ascribe any motivation to Redfield's words; even to this day, knowing that vaccinations began in December 2020, exactly as we had projected from the HHS time lines, I do not understand why he said it.

In that same interview and elsewhere, I was asked to clarify the inane comment that a mask was superior to a vaccine. Even the most devoted mask advocates, including news reporters, reacted with disbelief at such a notion. I did my best to cover for Redfield, but I absolutely needed to state the truth. "You know, Martha, I hate to comment on somebody else's statement, but that statement is just, I don't know where that statement comes from. I think it was taken out of context or maybe it was said inadvertently, but I don't think anyone believes that," I tried to explain. "I really don't think that Dr. Redfield believes that."

"He was very deliberate in his statement," McCallum noted, breaking in.

"I was going to say, I can't really comment on why people say certain things," I further replied. "We all make missteps when we speak."

Redfield's Congressional testimony on September 23 immediately caught my attention. I watched in disbelief as Redfield told Congress that "more than 90 percent of the population"—more than three hundred million people in the US—remains susceptible to the illness. The statement was based on incomplete and outdated data, as well as an apparent lack of understanding of the literature, and it struck me as one of the most erroneous and fear-inducing proclamations of any public health official to that moment. Approximately two hundred thousand Americans had already died from COVID; the last thing the public needed was an exaggeration of the future risks, implying to some that ten times that number could still die.

First of all, the numbers didn't add up. At that point, confirmed cases in the US already totaled approximately seven million, and the CDC itself had estimated that approximately ten times the number of confirmed cases, a very conservative estimate, were likely to have had the infection. A Stanford seropositivity study back in April had shown that confirmed cases underestimated the total infections by a factor of approximately forty times. It made no sense that only 9 percent, or thirty million Americans, had been infected.

Second, the 9 percent calculation was blatantly wrong. That number came from antibody testing by the states. I looked at the CDC website myself, and sure enough, the data was based on antiquated testing from several states. Some antibody totals were pulled from several months earlier, before many of those states had experienced a significant number of cases. It therefore grossly underestimated the number of cases that had already occurred. The data was simply not valid, but you needed to pay attention to the details.

More importantly, Redfield's basic claim was fundamentally flawed. The conclusion that serum antibody testing revealed the entire population of those protected from COVID was counter to an entire body of published literature and contrary to fundamental knowledge of immunology, including other coronavirus infections. It was well known that antibody tests showed one cross-section in time—they were transient—even though immune protection can last. From studies on SARS-2 and most other viruses, antibody levels change over a span of months. They typically appear in the first couple of weeks, peak in a few months, and then decrease over a span of several months.

The literature on COVID had already shown these patterns. A month before this press conference, a *Nature Reviews Immunology* study on COVID-19 explicitly stated, "The absence of specific antibodies in the serum does not necessarily mean an absence of immune memory," and explained, "memory B-cells and T-cells may be maintained even if there are not measurable levels of serum antibodies." Japan's study demonstrated this dramatically. In their study, antibody levels increased from 5.8 percent to 46.8 percent over the course of the summer. The most dramatic increase occurred in late June and early July, paralleling the rise in daily confirmed cases within Tokyo, which peaked on August 4. Out of the 350 individuals who completed both offered tests, 21.4 percent of those who tested negative became positive, and 12.2 percent of initially positive participants became negative for antibodies. A striking 81.1 percent of IgM-antibody-positive cases at first testing became negative in only one month. They stated that "[antibody tests] may significantly underestimate previous COVID-19 infections." It had also been widely reported in several major scientific journals that antibody responses are not necessarily detectable in all COVID patients, especially those with less severe forms.

But the flaws in Redfield's estimate extended deeper. Even those familiar with first-year college biology know that other components of the immune system, memory B-cell and T-cells, provide protection from virus infections. Some T-cells kill the virus, and they also help antibodies form. T-cells develop and provide protection that lasts far longer, even after antibodies disappear—sometimes for years in other SARS viruses. T-cells for this virus had already been documented, even in people unexposed to SARS-2, meaning that in these cases, cross-protection was present from T-cells originating in response to other coronaviruses. T-cells had also been found in individuals with completely asymptomatic SARS-2 infections. NIH Director Francis Collins had highlighted that very data in his *Director's Blog* a few weeks earlier, writing, "In fact, immune cells known as memory T cells also play an important role in the ability of our immune systems to protect us against many viral infections, including—it now appears—COVID-19."

Scientists from some of the top research institutions in the world, like Sweden's Karolinska Institute, San Diego's La Jolla Institute, Duke University, Berlin, and others had published this evidence. Karolinska demonstrated T-cell immunity in both asymptomatic and mild cases of COVID—even if antibody-negative.

Singapore researchers had noted robust T-cell responses to this virus, SARS2, from seventeen-year-old SARS1 samples. Since T-cells are obviously not discovered by antibody tests, those individuals were not included in Redfield's count. Yet he apparently had not considered this essential, indeed fundamental, point as he testified to Congress and made headlines.

After watching this debacle on TV, I knew full well what was coming later that day. The media would latch on to this and create even more public panic. I also knew that the responsibility for clarifying this grossly erroneous statement would be mine. There was no question it would come up at the president's press conference, and even if it did not, it still needed to be explained.

I rushed over to Derek Lyons's office to update him and to make sure we would alert the president beforehand. A few others in the West Wing were there, so I summarized to them what had been said to Congress. The mood ranged from amazement to dejection to frustration. An advisor to the president on legal matters warned me, with a smile on his face, "Scott, don't just bluntly say, 'Redfield is wrong!' Say something softer, like 'He misstated things.'"

I nodded, knowing that I needed to restrain my words, even though this was the same man who had tried to destroy me in the national press a few days earlier. But this wasn't personal at all. Clarifying the facts about the pandemic and countering the unending barrage of misinformation and pseudoscience about it, in this case coming from within the administration itself, was one of my most important roles in this national crisis.

During the pre-brief in the Oval Office a few hours later, I outlined the issue to the president. It was decided, as expected, that I would answer the question when it came up. And so it did. A reporter from ABC News directly asked me if Redfield's statement that more than 90 percent of Americans remained susceptible to the disease was true. I took the friendly advice I had received earlier in the day. "I think that Dr. Redfield misstated something there," I said, and then did my best to calmly explain the problems with outdated information and the contribution of cross-reactive T-cells and T-cell protection that would not have been included in his data. I correctly stated what was widely known and factual—that the protection from the virus "is not solely determined by the percent of people who have antibodies." During my answer, as I fended off interruptions, I tried to explain in understandable language as best I could.

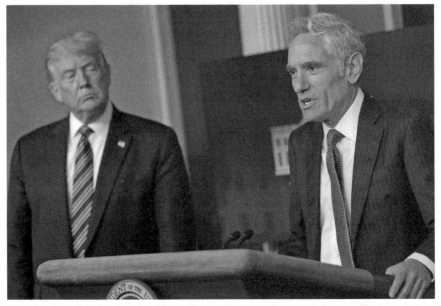

I attempted to clarify remarks from the podium to the press, always a challenge given the open hostility directed our way, while the president observed. (*Credit: Official White House photographers*)

I also made a serious effort to be somewhat delicate, because I felt extremely uncomfortable about having to correct the director of the CDC on the national stage.

Unfortunately, my disgust with the confrontational mood in that press room prevented me from being more diplomatic when that reporter asked, "Who are we to believe?" My reflexive answer was "You're supposed to believe in the science, and I am telling you the science." Then I referred him to several expert scientists by name. However, I had the strong sense that he was not really interested in the facts at all. Rather, it was another attempt to amplify discord.

After exiting the press room, I walked alongside the president. He briefly stopped to check the news coverage on the set of TV monitors outside the briefing room, as he typically chose to do. After some banter between the president and the staff standing in the area, we began walking back toward the Oval Office. President

Trump turned to me on his right, smiling wryly but with a genuinely puzzled look on his face. "Is Redfield political or just stupid?" he asked, subtly shaking his head. I looked right back at the president and hesitated. The answer was obvious to both of us.

Needless to say, the media immediately played up the disagreement between me and Redfield. It fed into their narrative of conflict between me and the other Task Force doctors, one that Redfield personally caused with his offensive and unwarranted remark that everything I said was "false." Later, Dr. Fauci appeared on TV and criticized my straightforward attempt to clarify important information as "extraordinarily inappropriate." I wondered if he was more concerned with protecting his bureaucrat colleague's reputation and undermining mine than ensuring that correct information was being told to the American public.

Martin Kulldorff, the world-renowned Harvard epidemiologist, posted his reaction on Twitter: "Scott Atlas stated the simple fact that immunity is higher than those with antibodies, whereupon Dr. Fauci criticizes him without contradicting what was actually said. Stating a simple scientific fact is not 'extraordinarily inappropriate.' What is going on?"

CHAPTER 11
"Don't Rock the Boat!"

Continuing her campus and state visits, Dr. Birx never stopped doling out her own policy recommendations. She and she alone was the representative of the Task Force to the governors and local officials from coast to coast, and her written words were the official advice from the White House. She always emphasized certain points—test and quarantine all positive tested students and all those exposed to them; close bars and restaurants; strictly limit groups; make sure everyone wears a mask, always and everywhere. And of course, continue all the standard mitigation measures.

I agreed about the standard mitigation measures—handwashing, extra sanitization standards, social distancing, and masks when you cannot be distant. I wrote it in op-eds, I stated it during my interviews, and whenever I had the chance I tried to add it into every presidential speech or briefing. I even explicitly began my part of the Task Force conference call with college presidents and administrators by reinforcing that message. The main difference was that I also pressed policies to increase protection of high-risk individuals as well as stop the damage from the Birx-Fauci lockdowns and their policies of isolating young, healthy, low-risk people.

But to Birx, it was always and only about stopping all cases, no matter the evidence that her policies failed to do so or the multiple harms they inflicted.

Her lack of discussion about the data relevant to policy harms should not have been a surprise, but it was frustrating. After all, their policies had grossly failed. The Task Force failed early in the pandemic to deploy the necessary testing, before the infection had spread so widely. The Task Force policies of lockdowns failed to save the known high-risk elderly from dying, even though nursing homes were already highly regulated and access was controllable. They even failed early on to warn Americans to take the pandemic seriously. Fauci had explicitly told the nation on January 29, 2020, that there was nothing to worry about, and on February 29 he said there was no need for social distancing. Ironically, the single most relevant statistic about the pandemic—excess mortality, i.e., deaths above and beyond what would have occurred naturally—was not mentioned, to my knowledge, until I presented it in the White House when discussing the relative performance of the US or individual states. A full eight months of death statistics had accumulated without any reference to the one universally known comparative tool to quantify results. And why not? I guess the reason for their ignorance was simply that none of them were epidemiologists... of course!

Birx had one game plan, and she stuck to it, regardless of the evidence of failure. She never once admitted that more could be done to save high-risk people when I suggested that—like other Task Force members—she balked at the notion that we could do more. Her advice for more general public mandates and restrictions, more quarantines, and more societal lockdowns was not just provided verbally on her dozens of visits to local officials, university administrators, and governors. She was also quoted extensively in the regional and national media, and everyone in the administration saw it. Her comments were highlighted in national news, and they were unavoidable throughout the West Wing, in every office, on the four-on-one monitors.

Birx's polices were enacted throughout the country, in almost every single state, for the entire pandemic—this cannot be denied; it cannot be deflected. As the traveling representative of the White House Coronavirus Task Force, Dr. Birx spoke about mandates and lockdowns, even when her statements directly conflicted with those of the president of the United States. No matter that his constant message was to augment the protection of the vulnerable but end the lockdowns, to reopen schools and society. It did not matter that her bar and restaurant restrictions and school closures were not backed by sound science. No matter that the president said in virtually every public statement that masks should be worn "when you cannot socially distance" rather than by everyone, everywhere. While serving in the name of the White House as Task Force coordinator, she effectively set and then disseminated national policy. And because her policies were those that were enacted on the ground, the success or failure of the pandemic management must necessarily rest on her policies, not on those who criticized what was enacted. Period.

And why did she speak contrary to the views of the president? What was going on, I asked Derek Lyons and John Rader? It was bizarre, in my mind, that the president was saying one thing while the White House Task Force representative was saying something entirely different, indeed contradictory. Wasn't it harmful for the administration's policy message to be so inconsistent? Wouldn't that create a lack of confidence in an already fearful public? And even though the governors were in charge of their own states' on-the-ground pandemic management, wasn't the correct policy advice the most important thing by far for the White House to voice to the nation?

Instead, no one ever set her straight on her role. The VP's chief of staff, Marc Short, confided in me more than once, "Scott, I was saying those things months ago. I am 100 percent in agreement with you. And I am living the school closures myself; it's horrible." Trump's COS Mark Meadows also told me several times that my views on the Birx-Fauci lockdowns and the failure of their policies were correct.

It didn't matter, though. When I asked how to handle questions about Birx's discordant advice, there was one consistent reply from both: "We agree, Scott...but we don't want to rock the boat." They were undoubtedly correct that for the president to challenge or fire

Birx would have created a huge story. She later confessed, after President Biden assumed office, that she, Fauci, and Redfield had a pact that they would resign together if one was replaced, as reported by the *New York Times*.

Still, I was frankly dumbstruck at the lack of leadership in the White House. These inner-circle staffers served a president who had shown no fear of upsetting others, to say the least. Yet the White House was held hostage to the anticipated reaction of Dr. Birx and its consequences in the media. The only person who offered a different reply to my query was Jared Kushner. I asked him what I should do while Birx was telling governors to increase restrictions, closures, and mandates, and to prolong the lockdowns, despite being opposite to what the president was saying to the press. His answer was always the same: "Talk to the vice president; he runs the Task Force." And he was right.

And what about her recommendations on the road? After telling Short, Meadows, and others to no avail that I had a couple of prominent governors chewing my ear off about Birx's ceaseless promotion of business closures, shutdowns of restaurants and schools, mask mandates, quarantining of healthy college students, and other restrictions, I finally recommended that they call the VP directly.

Birx herself openly admitted that some governors refused her visits, shaking her head as if they were acting in woeful ignorance. My take was the opposite—these governors understood from their own detailed analysis that the Birx-Fauci lockdowns were destroying communities and did not significantly alter the curves of cases and deaths. Yet her interpretation was "They are minimizing the seriousness of the virus," as if a desire to mitigate the severe harms of the lockdowns was somehow "denying the science."

Kushner made the obvious judgment at a COVID Huddle. Looking at one of Birx's state summary sheets, he eyed the data tabulated at the top and then the list of recommendations filling the bottom half. He politely suggested, "Let's eliminate the list of recommendations; they know what they're doing now, don't you think?" Governors were deep into running their own state policies.

We should just present the numbers—even though the tabulations were simply recycled data from the states themselves.

Unfortunately, nothing actually changed. Birx persisted in promoting her own advice: recommendations that prompted fear and perpetuated the lockdowns. And that advice was implemented by almost all the governors, regardless of any attempt to deny that and avoid accountability.

Eventually I figured out the dynamic. Birx obviously was very knowledgeable about two things, regardless of her expertise on the pandemic itself. First, she knew that the VP had her back, often echoing her words. Clearly, he was conscious that the Task Force—which he directed—was the most visible evidence of his own work in the administration. That meant that its perceived positives must be protected—nothing about it that the public viewed as positive would be minimized or criticized. Pence had zero intention of "rocking the boat" with Birx or Fauci, even though he was very receptive to my thoughts and readily agreed with the data I presented.

Second, Birx, having been in Washington for decades, understood something else that I certainly did not—how politicians worked. She was fully aware, unlike me, that there was no one who really had the guts to tell the truth to her or to the public. After all, an election was approaching.

*   *   *   *   *

My point—that we could *increase* protection of high-risk individuals—generated backlash, and not only from Birx. This was a sensitive spot for everyone on the Task Force, understandably, given that they had worked on the pandemic for seven months by the time I joined. Everyone was concerned with the death tallies; I never doubted that. But several in the Task Force, the VP included, became very defensive when I pushed for increasing protection of the elderly. The VP declared that they were already doing everything possible to protect the high-risk, the elderly, including in the nursing homes. Giroir claimed they could do no more, that they had developed and deployed a massive testing capacity; I concurred that they did well at developing the testing capacity. He and Seema Verma had successfully placed point-of-care testing in every nursing home; I agreed that was extremely important. Dr. Birx joined in trying to refute the whole notion of targeting more protection to those at risk to die. She strongly tried to reject my point, leaning across the table and emphatically telling me, "Nothing more could be done; we are already doing everything!" But stating something aggressively did not change the facts. Their efforts were failing to stop the deaths, and more *could* be done. Instead of thinking through my suggestions, their immediate response was to band together, to cover their collective behinds.

I wasn't explicitly criticizing their past efforts, but I disagreed. I challenged their notion that everything possible was being done. Why were we testing nursing home staff only once per week? We all knew that nursing home cases were almost always brought in by staff members. And many staff members worked in more than one nursing home, so that was an incredibly high-risk group to test. Why were we using the same broad recommendation on testing for all nursing homes—shouldn't we rapidly increase testing if the surrounding community, where the workers lived, had more cases? We already were tracking COVID visits to the ER in the communities. Why wasn't that simple measure being put to use strategically to protect seniors? After the Task Force's earlier failures on testing, they finally had an amazing testing capability; so why were we performing most tests in low-risk age groups, people under the age of sixty-five? I pointed out examples like LA County, where those eighteen to forty-nine, a low-risk age, made up 43 percent of the population but accounted for 66 percent of all the testing at that point in the early fall. Also, why were we ignoring seniors living on their own or in the community who were being exposed when they gathered in senior centers, where they had no testing? No, I insisted, much more could be done.

After voicing my concerns, one Task Force member did step forward. CMS's Seema Verma and I had separately developed a productive, ongoing dialogue. We worked together on a refined set of guidelines for nursing homes and jointly recommended far more frequent point-of-care testing in residential settings for seniors. We stressed the importance of increasing the frequency of staff testing to three times per week or more, if community spread was high. We added the criterion "COVID-like-illness to the emergency department" to determine community infection levels, since that was simpler, already being tabulated everywhere, and didn't suffer from the arbitrary nature of testing. I worked with Seema and Brad Smith of domestic policy to explore adding alerts of community activity to high-risk seniors living independently who were already known to Medicare. Seema also added new incentives to performance and instituted partnerships for improving protection control with neighboring hospitals. I personally reported every state with increasing CLI activity directly to her, and she then communicated that alert to the nursing homes in those regions of the country. I worked hard with Ja'Ron Smith, deputy director of the Office of American Innovation, and others to prioritize millions of tests to high-risk faculty members at HBCUs.

These were excellent working relationships, and yes, more was done to improve the protection of the elderly and other high-risk individuals. And was that increased protection to the elderly successful? While many factors certainly helped, the data speaks for itself—as was proven months later, our measures helped reduce nursing home COVID mortality from April's 21 percent to about half that by the time I left in November.

CHAPTER 12
Inside the COVID Huddle

COVID Huddles were working meetings specifically intended to set the focus for the entire communications effort from the White House about the pandemic—events, presidential speeches, and interview themes and talking points. Kushner usually ran the COVID Huddles, unless he was out of town. These were held in the historic Roosevelt Room in the West Wing, approximately three times per week. After initially hiding me in his office and placing the meeting on speakerphone so I could listen, Kushner told me to attend these meetings, and I soon understood why. These were far more than just political strategy meetings. The COVID Huddles were designed to be messaging meetings, and the context was political strategy, not policy. In practice, it was not possible to separate the policy from the communication.

This regularly held meeting was where most of those representing the Executive Branch charged with interfacing with the media and the public received their updates about the status of the pandemic—and that update was always directly from Dr. Birx, the Task Force Coordinator. The communications strategy would derive from the data she presented, and from her policy prescriptions.

There was a second element to the communications effort that confounded me. In my assessment, almost everything from the communications side of the White House was reactive rather than proactive. The output from this meeting was primarily based on their anticipation of the political reaction. I never really understood that until much later, and it frustrated me—weren't we supposed to put forth the correct policy? I was extremely naive, in retrospect, but I never accepted that this was political; for me, the pandemic management had nothing to do with politics. Once I grasped the political motivation dominating everyone else, though, it made me even more determined to fight for the best policies to stop the death and destruction. As usual, I was an outlier.

Aside from Kushner, Adam Boehler (Kushner's former college roommate), Birx, and their staffs, a large and very heterogeneous group attended the COVID Huddles, later entitled "China Virus Huddles" on the printed agendas. The list of attendees included high-level staff like HHS's Paul Mango with detailed knowledge about the status of vaccine and drug development, and others working on the logistics of new tests. These were competent, behind-the-scenes people without overwhelming egos, and I worked well with them during my months in Washington. John Rader, a Kushner advisor, and Staff Secretary Derek Lyons, to me the best critical thinkers in the West Wing, were also usually there. At the opposite extreme were purely political advisers who had almost no knowledge about the pandemic. Some were the most visible faces on TV, intimate counselors of the president on a host of issues. This group was there to get background but also to weigh in on the strategic plans for communicating on behalf of the administration.

Separate from these two groups were most of the communications team. Although Mark Meadows and Kayleigh McEnany never attended, and Stephen Miller only occasionally sat in, Hope Hicks typically did. She stood out for her decisiveness and clarity of thought. Hope was a highly capable interpreter of the discussion, frequently formulating the bottom line without much hesitancy and quickly devising key campaign events for the weeks ahead. In my mind, others in attendance, mainly the young communications team, were there to take direction. They often seemed overwhelmed—but they were just doing their best to help the president, looking for direction out of the hodgepodge of statements expressed in that room, in order to formulate their own talking points. With the level of hostility in the media that awaited, that was no minor undertaking.

I was sympathetic to them, not just because they were always battling the media. I realized that once I joined, everything became more difficult, more confusing. Instead of blindly accepting Dr. Birx's assessments, I often challenged what had previously been accepted as a given, and I had detailed data to back me up. This disrupted the status quo that had been present for months. I sensed that I was also an unwanted disruption to the entourage that followed Birx around. I began to suspect that they were part of the group likely running to the media to disparage me by feeding distortions of my words, as they were noticeably loyal to Birx.

It ultimately dawned on me that this meeting was, in many ways, more important than the Task Force meetings. Task Force meetings were for the most part operational updates, but the medical discussions were never directly on the president's radar. The COVID Huddle was more specifically for the White House, and it incorporated all of the president's key communicators. Here is where the policy met the communications strategy. It was a bit like watching the sausage being made; given that I was inherently negative about politics, this was not pleasant to sit through. For me, it was another source of frustration. Yet again, my task was to unwind the stream of misinformation being told to a medically naive group. In that regard, it was very similar to the Task Force!

Each meeting began with Kushner taking the lead on the short printed agenda, as always trying to be superconcise and setting a businesslike tone by first asking for a quick update from Birx. Based on what she reported at these meetings, they naturally assumed her interpretations of the success of the mandates, as well as the need to test healthy people and quarantine those testing positive, represented the consensus on "the science." From her opinions, their own media appearances and interview talking points were shaped. From Birx's descriptions and warnings about massive deaths if lockdowns were not enacted came the responses, like stressing more and more testing of healthy low-risk students, for instance, and the planning about events at the White House and on the road.

Few questioned the assertions of Dr. Birx at the COVID Huddles, mainly because virtually no one else in the room had any medical or science background whatsoever. That medical background was not the only thing that mattered, though. The truly essential ingredients were critical thinking and time to look at the data. Even if people were skeptical, and several confided to me that they had been for quite a while, most in the room were not analyzing the data—they had no time. Since Birx was the source of all the data that anyone heard, it was difficult for them to question it. They had other jobs, and they were focused on their own tasks.

Almost no one in the COVID Huddle truly grasped that the Birx strategy was not merely a failure at stopping the cases—it was far worse than that. The elderly kept dying and a massive health disaster was unfolding from the lockdown. Uninfected people were dying directly because of the closure of other medical care and their fear of seeking it. Meanwhile, kids were being sacrificed, and families were being utterly destroyed from severe economic hardships, translating into drug abuse, spousal abuse, child abuse, and a host of other harms.

One more oddity of the situation was never really verbalized until I forced the topic—the Birx lockdowns directly conflicted with the president's stated strategy of reopening schools and society while focusing on protecting the most vulnerable. That internal messaging discordance was destructive, not just personally frustrating. Meadows and others sometimes dismissed differences between me and Birx or the others as "the doctors disagree," as if the data did not matter, as if setting the correct policy was not the goal. The common theme I heard over the three months leading up to the election was pure politics—they didn't want to "rock the boat." They said they feared "upsetting" Birx, because she was held in high esteem by the public and "we were so close to an election," as Meadows and others kept reminding me. I wondered at times why even they asked me there.

Most people said nothing about the conclusions leading to the policies being advocated by Birx at these meetings. They simply accepted her conclusions. This was understandable—she had been the sole person in the room with any medical background for months prior to my arrival. The COVID Huddle group had no medical or science background and were there solely to be guided about messaging. However, a small number of people at these meetings occasionally expressed doubt, some more politely than others and usually outside the room, about the lack of sophistication of her tabulations. One particularly outspoken member of the COVID Huddle would tell me that there was nothing useful, indeed nothing that would merit the term "analysis." A few others were overtly aligned with me from the earliest days of my arrival. They were convinced that my interpretation and strategy of focusing protection to save the high-risk individuals while opening society would save more lives, and the Fauci-Birx strategy of locking down businesses and schools and quarantining healthy people was harmful and lacked common sense.

Most of these feelings were discussed in private, owing to the sensitivity about disagreeing with Dr. Birx. Even if they did not accept her views on the pandemic, nearly everyone was reluctant to alienate her. I later came to understand that this dynamic had a historical context. When the president and Fauci had significant disagreements that became public many months before I arrived, those present considered the arrival of Birx, relatively speaking, as a breath of fresh air. At least she was not as overtly contrary as Fauci, they explained. That timing also correlated with the VP taking over leadership of the Task Force, although I was told that Pence himself did not make the addition of Birx to the team. And some had already seen her volatile behavior in the past. I was told several stories about her interrupting all who challenged her, and I saw this behavior myself in both the Task Force and COVID Huddle meetings. After the initial instances, I learned to calmly admonish her discourteous interruptions with a stern "please let me finish" before continuing.

Given that Kushner asked me to advise on the pandemic, and further insisted that I attend these specific meetings, he obviously understood the dilemma. But Birx reported to the vice president, and not to Kushner or anyone else. When I would tell Kushner that I had to deal with hostile, screaming governors complaining about the messages from Birx on her visits to their states, he usually answered, "That's the responsibility of the vice president. Tell Pence." Unfortunately, the VP and his chief of staff, Marc Short, decided that upsetting Birx was simply not worth the risk to the upcoming election. Short even cautioned me to avoid raising the issue. Birx was not to be touched, period.

Ultimately, a couple of governors simply refused to allow her to visit—even when the VP's office itself called to arrange visits. That said, some in the vice president's staff understood that Birx was both wrong and often contradicted policy recommendations of the administration. I was told that directly, repeatedly, by several people at the highest levels. Others at the COVID Huddles also understood the data on their own—Lyons, Rader, and Hope Hicks all showed that critical thinking, not an MD education, was the only essential "credential" to figure out what was happening. Despite that, the White House, the VP, and the messaging kept dancing to the tune of Birx, specifically because she was spouting the narrative most accepted by the mass media.

I didn't care about political risk, though. I couldn't have cared less about the personal feelings of anyone in the White House. The policies recommended by Birx and Fauci had been implemented by almost every state, and those policies were empirically failing. For me, the only thing that counted was to communicate the correct policy, to stop the deaths and destruction. Someone had to step up and speak the truth.

* * * * *

Regardless of my presence in the press briefings, at the contentious Task Force meetings, or at the COVID Huddles, Birx remained the main advisor and the only Task Force representative to governors. Hers was the only output in writing to states, and she doled it out to every single state in the nation. Until I arrived, no one had challenged anything she said during her six months as the Task Force Coordinator.

She also was key to educating everyone at the COVID Huddles. I had expected complex analyses of special data that others had no access to, but the trends that Birx put forth to the White House communicators, day after day, meeting after meeting, were fundamentally simple tabulations of weekly tallies. Adding to the problem, Birx invoked circular reasoning as "proof" that locking down was successful in stopping the spread of cases. Like so many others during the pandemic, she relied on models that predicted a certain number of cases and deaths without any accounting for the cyclical decrease in cases that characteristically occurred as time went on, due to increasing immunity, seasonality, and other factors. Because those continued high levels predicted by her model-of-choice failed to materialize, lo and behold, it must have been due to the success of the interventions in place!

To have more impact, to convey the lessons from what we had learned about risk directly to the public, I decided on a new strategy. I needed to show accurate charts and explain the true trends to everyone in the Huddles, especially the communications folks. These people were designing communications and events for the president and appeared before the cameras themselves. I kept reminding myself that it was not productive to argue with Dr. Birx or anyone else on the Task Force—that was destined to fail anyway. The key was to communicate the truth to the American public, I kept stressing, and the president's statements must reflect accurate data, even if I could not get through to Birx and the Task Force.

At several COVID Huddles, I showed detailed charts documenting the true dates of deaths or cases. I took time to show the actual data, the discrepancies between trends shown by Birx and the accurate trends from Arizona, Florida, Texas, and elsewhere—a detailed analysis often provided by some outstanding analysts outside the government. These illustrated in detail how the reported dates of deaths were at times tallying deaths from weeks or months prior. In turn, newly accurate assignment of dates changed the entire shape of the trend curve. That meant peaks on charts were off by weeks, so if one designed a policy to the peak, or concluded an impact of a policy from the decline of a peak, it would be incorrect. Whenever I could catch him, I showed Kushner similar charts of trends, evidence on the impact of lockdowns, case surges through mask mandates—and he usually nodded his head, saying, "I know, I know, you're right," as he rushed to another important meeting about political strategy.

After the COVID Huddles, I also began to run upstairs to the communications team offices, adjacent to Kayleigh's office, to show Alyssa Farah and Brian Morgenstern and their team what was happening. I thought it was critical to have the communications team see the evidence, printed on pages, so they knew why I was saying what I was saying. Shouldn't everyone who communicated to the public be informed about the truth? I learned to walk literally everywhere with my laptop case overflowing with charts, articles, and the latest printouts of data, eliminating any possibility of carrying my computer itself.

At the COVID huddles, I tried to make the team aware of my fundamental difference with what was being communicated to the country. With rare exceptions, the nation was implementing exactly what Birx and Fauci and the Task Force had recommended. I tried to frame my basic thinking many times to anyone who would listen: We know who is at risk, and there are two alternatives. We could lock down everyone so the vulnerable are *indirectly* protected, or we could do everything to protect them *directly* but let low-risk people live their lives. I explained that we needed to do more to directly protect those who we knew could die, because they were not being protected. I kept stressing that locking down, restricting everyone, was extraordinarily harmful, especially to the working class and the poor. The lockdowns were a luxury of the rich, and it was unconscionable to continue them.

Data on the Birx-Fauci lockdown harms was piling up, and I was frantic that it was being ignored by those in charge. Meanwhile my inbox was filling up with hundreds of emails from regular people—mostly Americans but some across the globe—describing in excruciating detail the human cost of the lockdowns. This was a true catastrophe. In my mind, this was not special knowledge but common sense; it should not have been necessary to say it. It was also evident in the data, numbers that I had written and recited more than a dozen times. But after sitting in with the Task Force and hearing the COVID Huddles, I was thrilled, almost shocked, whenever someone took me aside and confided that they agreed with me. I remember asking Hope Hicks once if she had a background in science, after she explained very logically that she understood the rationale I espoused about opening while increasing protection of the vulnerable. She laughed at my question, probably because she, too, thought it was obvious, common sense.

I never fully understood why there was no admission, even internally by the Task Force, that the Birx-Fauci strategy did not work. I knew the media was incredibly receptive to their views—after all, it fit so nicely with their anti-Trump narrative. Disagreeing with Trump, especially in this election year, ensured near idolatry on cable TV and in the *New York Times* or *Washington Post*. But I never thought politics was the main driver of those on the Task Force. Perhaps it was an unstated fear that they were in way too deep to admit their errors. They certainly had plenty of backing from the public health establishment, many of whom were also acting out of self-protection.

But the cases still spread, and the lockdowns still failed to protect the elderly. How could there be no recognition that nursing home deaths made up 30, 40, even 80 percent of deaths in some states while the lockdown was destroying everyone else.

Birx often pushed back when I said it was not a sensible goal to "stop all cases of COVID at all costs." She explained, "We know from the data that cases lead to hospitalizations, and hospitalizations lead to deaths." I would reply, "Yes, of course we know that. But we cannot stop all cases. That is also already proven. Tens of millions of Americans already have had the virus. We cannot even stop all deaths; that is naive. But we can and *must* increase the protection of those at risk to die. Only a narrow group has a significant risk to die, not everyone. What we can do is minimize the deaths, that's the entire point—to stop people from dying. And we should stop sacrificing children and destroying families by locking down healthy, low-risk people."

Only later would journals publish studies like one in January 2021 from Stanford University's infectious disease scientists and epidemiologists Bendavid, Oh, Bhattacharya, and Ioannidis that showed the mitigating impact of the extraordinary measures used in almost every state was not significant and, according to the study's senior author, Ioannidis, usually harmful, even "pro-contagion." That was validated by Agrawal's study in June 2021, who found that deaths were falling before lockdowns were imposed, but once lockdowns were instituted, the death toll began rising.

* * * * *

One Friday, in late October, I received not one but two emails that left me feeling overwhelmed at the outpouring of support from people suffering under the lockdowns. One was from someone who had written me several times, expressing gratitude and support for my speaking out. As the wife of a doctor and an avid reader about the pandemic, she had sent email after email, encouraging me for weeks. She wrote about how it "made (her) blood boil" that CNN was criticizing me for not being qualified, as their own medical experts and journalists "pontificated" about COVID, without any knowledge whatsoever. She had been so kind, clearly worried about me taking so much media abuse.

And then, one afternoon, she wrote, "Dr. Atlas, I want to talk to you about something you have brought up a million times at least, about the dangers of lockdowns. It certainly hit home for me last Friday. My beloved husband…took his life while we were on vacation…. His depression started when COVID-19 started and the lockdowns began."

Horrified, I continued reading. "I just want you to know how right you have been about everything and I hope you will continue your crusade against lockdowns. If it helps one family to not go through what we are experiencing, it would be a victory."

I started crying, standing there. This was not acceptable. This was sinful, counter to the public good, an abuse of public health.

Public health leaders were recommending policies that were killing people with these insane lockdowns.

Two hours later, I received another email of support, one of dozens that I received every day. But this one was different. It began, "I wanted to write you a letter sending my appreciation and gratitude for representing citizens enduring the collateral damage of lockdown policies. I hope you will treat this information as confidential since we are keeping this news private. My family is the collateral damage. My 14-year-old daughter…made a serious attempt to end her life. Thankfully, she was not successful and we are trying hard to convince her to live."

It was too much for me. To sit in that Task Force, to listen to these so-called experts, with such influence, people who denied the data, who were not even critiquing the scientific literature. People who hadn't worked with patients for decades, who showed no perspective on clinical medicine. Public health officials who heinously and consistently disregarded the horrible destruction occurring in the wake of *their* policies—policies that were undeniably followed throughout the country, no matter what they claimed otherwise, no matter what the president or anyone else tried to say. The lockdowns—*their lockdowns*—were at this point, in my mind, reprehensible, totally unforgivable, a crime against humanity.

I felt sick inside. I had to tell someone. I contacted some friendly faces right away in the White House, telling them what I had received—Johnny McEntee, John Rader, a couple of others. I was distraught, enraged, totally disgusted with the nonscientific calls for locking down.

I grabbed my briefcase and started heading out, intending to walk toward my usual exit from the West Wing, past the Rose Garden, out the East Wing, and down Pennsylvania Avenue to my hotel. But I stopped myself. I turned back, climbed the stairs and walked to the office area of the communications team. No one was there except Brian Morgenstern, deputy press secretary. Brian was a hard worker who did his best to navigate the constant chaos of interfacing with the media as a representative of the Trump White House. Brian was a key member of the communications team attending the

COVID Huddle. He had seen my disagreements many times, and I presumed he was often conflicted—that was part of the problem, the lack of clarity from those in charge.

It didn't matter who was there, though. I was beside myself. I barged in, angrily told him about the emails that I had received and exploded in rage. "Those policies of lockdown are killing people! Do you understand that?? Do you understand this is not a game— these lockdowns are destroying people?? Do you understand that?!" I demanded. Brian looked at me, stunned. He replied, calmly, "Yes, Dr. Atlas, I understand. I am so sorry." I turned around and left the White House in tears.

To this day, I cannot understand why the human cost of the lockdowns never mattered to anyone else on the Task Force. It was never brought up while I was there, not a single doctor ever spoke of it. The media continues to ignore perhaps the most remarkable insight in the Fauci email trove discovered under FOIA in June 2021—the total lack of mention of harms from the lockdown throughout the pandemic. But I never seriously considered shutting up. That was my whole reason for coming to Washington, my entire motivation. And I kept hearing these pleas and personal tragedies every single day. No matter what happened at these meetings, I was not going to stop fighting for the millions of Americans who were bearing the brunt of the lockdowns and suffering unconscionable physical and psychological harms that will last for decades.

*   *   *   *   *

I had come to the point of dreading it when I received another Task Force email invitation from the VP's staff. By now, I was 100 percent convinced of the futility of the Task Force meetings. I had already repeated the evidence about cases, the efficacy comparisons of lockdown versus no lockdown, the problems with the inaccuracy of trends, the fallacies about schools, and the destruction of the lockdowns until I was blue in the face, even at the COVID Huddles.

At the end of another long stretch of assertions about correlations relying on pseudoscience, I had had enough. I was mentally burned out. I had no energy left to voice my obvious disagreement, so I remained silent. As the meeting ended, I returned with my cookie and cappuccino in hand to John Rader's office, hoping to find a sympathetic ear. I related one of the many inane episodes to him. He then asked, "So what did you say?" I looked up and told him. "Nothing. I couldn't bring myself to say the same thing again." John was irritated, a rarity for him. "Scott, never, never do that. If you disagree, you must speak up. Say it. Otherwise, it sits there, left unchallenged." I knew he was right, and I promised to do that next time.

It came soon that I had the opportunity to fulfill my duty to speak the truth. At the next COVID Huddle, Dr. Birx went through her set of charts, explaining how "we stopped the spread of cases" in this state and that state. Then she repeated her earlier warning that if the spread was not stopped, that over 2 million Americans would die at this rate. She had learned nothing and was still relying on outdated, discredited theories that everyone was equally susceptible and that somehow cases would continue on a certain trajectory. She simply ignored what the data cycles had shown all over the world—declining cases over two to three months due to increasing immunity and a seasonal impact.

At the end, I slowly raised my hand and made a simple pronouncement. "I completely disagree." That was it. Nothing more. I had no more energy left to explain how misguided and harmful her policies were. Lockdowns were killing people, destroying millions of families and children, in this obsessive desire to stop a virus that was deadly only to the high-risk. And no one seemed to care.

*   *   *   *   *

It wasn't just health policy and clinical medical perspective that the Task Force doctors lacked. Testing was a topic that was actively mentioned at the Task Force, separate from the fiasco of the changing CDC guidance. Mentioning testing, though, is very different from tackling the more complex issues about PCR testing and cycle thresholds. Those were never noted at any Task Force meeting, other than by me.

It goes without saying that determining if someone is contagious is the fundamental reason for testing. The overwhelming majority of positive PCR tests, though, show virus fragments in people who are not contagious. This fact was widely known and reported in great detail in scientific studies as well as in newspapers by the time I arrived in Washington. That meant that most tests, using the extremely sensitive techniques in place, were detecting dead virus or such minute quantities of virus that a positive test was worse than meaningless: it was miscategorizing someone as contagious, thereby necessitating home confinement, isolation, and even quarantining others around them. This pitfall—a sensitivity so high that the test was essentially detecting false positives—was widely known to every person closely following the pandemic, because that technical problem was contributing greatly to the wrong policy actions. At that time, I was not aware that Dr. Fauci had stated in a July interview, before I arrived, the scientific truth about most PCR tests being performed. "At a cycle threshold of 35 or more, the chances of it being replication-competent [contagious] are miniscule...You gotta say it's just dead nucleotides, period."

Yet, the White House Task Force doctors sitting in the Situation Room for months—Birx, Fauci, Giroir, Redfield—literally never discussed this critical error during the meetings I sat through in Washington. They never mentioned it, not even after I distributed the research at a Task Force meeting in September. I remember making sure that everyone at the table had the data, along with supplemental papers by world-class epidemiologists and a summary document about the overall issues on PCR tests in this pandemic, while noting with a tinge of sarcasm, "I thought some people might actually be interested in reading the science."

Honestly, it didn't surprise me at all that there was never a minute's worth of discussion on this highly important issue. By September, I had no expectation of any sophisticated thinking from the Task Force doctors. But what stunned and saddened me was the realization that the Task Force had not thought critically about the specifics of testing in this pandemic. From my first days sitting in Jared's office listening to the Huddles by telephone, nothing about the pitfalls and erroneous conclusions derived from PCR testing was voiced. It was all about volume. How could it be that no one noted the difference between a positive PCR test and contagiousness? How could no one even mention the limitations with contact tracing for a virus that had already become widespread, having infected tens of millions of Americans, a virus that spread rapidly and silently? Why was this not a topic of discussion, regardless of the ultimate opinion?

That was all part of the puzzle of the Task Force doctors. There was a lack of scientific rigor in meetings I attended. I never saw them question the data. The striking uniformity of opinion by Birx, Redfield, Fauci, and Giroir was not anything like what I had seen in my career in academic medicine, and I took that as an absence of independent thought. And that's not science.

* * * * *

The inexplicable lack of critical thinking among the Task Force doctors, even after nine months, was hammered home in late September, when I was asked by the VP to prepare a presentation about testing for the Task Force. The VP invoked one of his favorite phrases—"iron sharpens iron"—and said that someone else (it was either Fauci or Birx) would also give an opinion. To me, this was ridiculous. After nine months, the Task Force still did not have total and complete knowledge about something so basic? I had zero inclination to provide this useless report, but I politely said, "Fine," to the VP's request.

After the meeting, as usual, I dropped in on Rader and Derek Lyons down the hall in the West Wing. Shaking my head in disgust, I explained that even a full nine months after the pandemic began, these "experts" still had no solid understanding of the strategy or rationale for testing. The idea that an explanation was still needed at this juncture was beyond absurd. Later, I wrote to the VP's staff in frustration, declining to produce the report, saying that I had no energy or interest in teaching basic information to people who after nine months on the Task Force still lacked such fundamental knowledge.

The idea of my giving a tutorial did not come up again. And that became my final Task Force meeting.

CHAPTER 13
POTUS Meets the Real Experts...in Secret

At this point, Dr. Birx's view of the pandemic was the established view for most in the White House, including the members of the communications team. She was the established authority in the eyes of the large group of nonmedical people involved in the thrice-weekly COVID Huddle held in the Roosevelt Room of the West Wing. She had a loyal following of mid- and lower-level staff surrounding her. No one doubted that she worked hard, traveling frequently to states and compiling numbers for months. But she had been the only person with any medical background in the room for months, so most naturally deferred to her.

Dr. Birx held court at the COVID Huddle, comfortable speaking to the nonmedical group in the meetings, pushing policies without being challenged, including testing healthy people, quarantining asymptomatic children and adults, and arbitrarily closing restaurants and bars, specifically "after 11:00 p.m." No one bothered to ask about the science behind that seemingly magical moment. Why not 9:30 p.m. or 11:30 p.m. or even 2:00 a.m.? What about the research that showed only a small fraction of cases stemming from bars and restaurants? Contact tracing data showed that only a tiny percentage of cases originated in restaurants and bars. That was ignored. In fact, it seemed completely unknown in the White House until I presented it.

Once I joined the discussions, predictably, the result was an internal policy conflict. Each state controlled its own policies, and almost all were locking down, mandating masks and closing schools, just as Dr. Birx wanted. I was exasperated at what I saw *inside* the White House, though. Shouldn't the administration at least try to first become thoroughly familiar with the research and analyze the data in order to devise public policy, then try to sway governors? And shouldn't the president's views prevail over those of Dr. Birx? Why was I here anyway?

* * * * *

After a couple of weeks, the disconnect between the Oval Office and the rest of the White House had become severe. The president needed to understand, as quickly as possible, that some of the country's leading experts disagreed with Dr. Birx's recommendations and that the data backed up his commonsense notion that the lockdowns were destroying the country.

I had some trepidation as to how to proceed. I had a gut feeling that, despite my warm welcome, academic expertise was not valued highly by this White House that prided itself on populism and distrust of technocratic elites. "I know a lot of smart doctors who say different things," Kushner once told me. While I am sure that was true, I nevertheless took that to mean something broader. To me, being an MD was not nearly sufficient to having expert-level knowledge. To many others, including some in the White House, a postgraduate degree after a name meant just that, even a government bureaucrat masquerading as one.

Regardless, the president needed to hear from true experts—physicians and other scientists who were independent researchers of national stature, who had conducted and published their own analyses outside of any bureaucratic or government position. It was also obvious to me that the American public would benefit from seeing the president seek a broader range of expert opinion.

Selfishly, perhaps, I also wanted to make sure people inside the White House as well as the public understood that I wasn't winging it. Everything I said was firmly based on the data. That wasn't even questionable, despite the absurd hit pieces in the media. Further, my strategy—the logical one of adding protection for those at high risk while reopening schools and low-risk activities—was accepted by many top health-policy experts and scientists across the country. The media's ideologically driven narrative declared the opposite. Mainstream outlets confidently asserted there was a universal consensus among public-health experts that lockdowns were essential, that the virus required total lockdown, and that those lockdowns would stop all COVID cases. These assertions were at best extremely naive and, at worst, unabashed lies.

It was also clear that the vice president needed to meet with scientists and doctors who held the outside perspective. It wasn't only that he ran the Task Force and, one would think, had the capacity to guide the discussion and state the bottom line. Personality-wise, the vice president was by nature overly complimentary and respectful to a fault. This meant that he was reflexively deferential to Drs. Fauci, Birx, and Redfield.

Dr. Birx, in particular, seemed to adore working with the vice president. She glowed from his every compliment. Always positive and professional, he handed her many. The two of them often worked together on visits to states, emphasizing her message and, thus, disregarding the fact that it was often contrary to the president's preferred policies that he voiced repeatedly. This was an established team, no doubt.

Since the president did not attend a single Task Force meeting, it's possible that her counsel didn't regularly make it to him. But the vice president must have understood that the president's views on reopening were incompatible with the advice coming out of the Task Force. This was the problem: the vice president had never been given any reason to doubt anything said by the medical constituents at the table. He had never been presented with data contrary to what they offered. He had never heard from people with medical knowledge other than from the self-selected handful in the Situation Room. My voice alone was not going to be enough.

Because I had been discussing the data and issues surrounding the pandemic for many months, I had a long list of experts at my fingertips to invite to the White House. My priority was adding authorities with the highest credibility in all the key areas, medical scientists who also knew how to articulate the reality about the data in succinct, straightforward terms. No one likes too much detail, and the president certainly did not want anything resembling a lecture. I also assumed that time would be very limited.

* * * * *

In early August, I approached my Stanford colleague Jay Bhattacharya, an expert in infectious disease, health policy, and economics, and told him I wanted to organize a private roundtable meeting with the president. I wanted the president to receive advice from nationally recognized academic experts.

Jay and I agreed that the meeting should focus on several key issues: 1) alleviating fear by conveying to the American public the true mortality numbers and the low risk to most people; 2) finally prioritizing resources to protect the high-risk vulnerable; and 3) ending lockdowns and letting everyone else get back to normal life. I stressed that we must keep highlighting the specific data on the destruction from the lockdown, the serious harms to public health, and the enormous harms of school closures.

I also revealed to Jay that I was already advocating internally for more specific, more aggressive moves, beyond the standard mitigation strategies, to make sure we increased protection of the vulnerable, including more testing of nursing-home staff, more protective equipment and testing at senior centers, and more proactive outreach to independent seniors. Jay offered fantastic information about existing mechanisms to identify high-risk seniors who lived in the community. We also kicked around ideas for other invitees. Meanwhile, he booked his flight to Washington.

I also expressed my desire to add people outside Stanford. The credibility of the discussion would be heightened and the views would be more thought-provoking if we had experts from other institutions.

After we hung up, I immediately began to assemble the group. By now, I understood that every background detail would be viciously attacked. After getting turned down by an excellent Stanford infectious disease scientist due to his fear of reprisal, I decided to move to the more important, non-Stanford world.

I first contacted Harvard's Martin Kulldorff, a brilliant authority on statistical analysis of infections and vaccines who was also a consultant to the FDA and the CDC, and gave him my interpretation of the data and what I thought were the appropriate policies to move ahead. He listened intently and agreed with my analysis. I asked whether he would be willing to share his views directly with the president, and he immediately said yes.

I then contacted Joe Ladapo, an associate professor of medicine and policy expert at UCLA. I had read his compelling op-eds about the pandemic, and we were both on email lists about the lockdown in California. Cody Meissner, chief of Pediatric Infectious Disease at Tufts School of Medicine, was next on my list. Cody is an authority on childhood infections and vaccines, and previously served as a CDC consultant. My calls with Joe and Cody were filled with enthusiasm. They grasped the importance of the situation and were thrilled by the once-in-a-lifetime opportunity to speak directly with the president of the United States.

I presented the roundtable idea to my friends John Rader and Derek Lyons. They both thought it was fantastic. I hand delivered a one-page prospectus to Kushner. I also ran it by Hope Hicks. After a few days, the roundtable had been approved by the key decision-makers. Go time!

On Monday, August 17, I messaged Jay: "It's on! Private roundtable with the President. On Wednesday. More to follow." I then reached out to Martin, Joe, and Cody to share the news. Plane tickets were purchased, and personal calendars rearranged. This would be a turning point. Or so I thought.

Three hours later, the roundtable was canceled via email by the vice president's scheduling office. I asked around and was informed that Dr. Birx would have been traveling at the same time. There was concern in the West Wing that, as a result, the roundtable would have been interpreted as an attempt to undermine her. I was disappointed, but I understood, agreeing the media would have leapt at the chance to sow discord and diminish its importance.

At the same time, I realized it would have been very uncomfortable for Dr. Birx—a potential disaster, in truth. Birx bristled whenever she was challenged by me. I later learned that was not new behavior, nor was it a reaction unique to me.

The individuals I had invited knew the data cold. They understood the damage from the lockdowns. Dr. Birx would have suddenly found herself in the minority among a group of respected authorities. But the information needed to be heard by the president and the vice president, even if it would make people uncomfortable.

* * * * *

Over the next few days, I felt uneasy, uncertain that the meeting would be rescheduled at all. I detected a lack of interest by those who controlled calendars. I spoke with Kushner, Hicks, and several others, pressing the need to hold the roundtable. I made a case that the president would benefit: he would gain credibility by openly "listening to the scientists." I displayed, again, the impeccable résumés of the prospective participants. I also once more insisted that it was imperative for the vice president to attend. After a few more days, everyone finally agreed to move ahead. We rescheduled for August 26, when everyone knew Dr. Birx would also be able to attend.

The White House communications team became more involved, planning for a potential live Q and A with the press during the roundtable. Information was distributed several days in a row at the COVID Huddle, thereby making it visible to Dr. Birx and dozens of others. I helped prepare a fact sheet, complete with talking points and the bios of the participants. I went over the details again with the communications team. Edits were made. A list of talking points was drafted and finalized. We then turned to the venue. The Cabinet Room was considered at first, but the Oval Office was chosen.

Everything was set. Then things began to unravel again. As the date approached, I was notified that the vice president would be unable to attend. He would be traveling to give his acceptance speech for the nomination. OK, but it was crucial for the head of the Task Force to meet these experts. I convinced the vice president's staff to squeeze in a meeting the following day. Of course, the four invited participants didn't need to be convinced of the need to remain in Washington for an additional twenty-four hours. All scrambled to accommodate the abrupt change.

On August 25, the day before the rescheduled roundtable, Dr. Birx sent out an email stating that she would not attend. She did not say she had a conflict, simply that it would "not be good" for her to do so. I thought back to all the times Kushner had assured me, "Birx is all about helping the president," she is "100-percent MAGA," and "a team player." Hardly, I thought, judging from this reaction.

That same morning, I was abruptly called to Kushner's office. He told me the roundtable would not occur at all, mumbling something about the president's schedule. I was stunned. I knew about Dr. Birx's email.

I strongly protested the decision. I reiterated the importance of the president and vice president hearing from a group of independent and nationally known experts. I also thought the event would demonstrate to the public in a highly visible and meaningful way that the president was directly engaged, and further, that his opponents' claims about him "not listening to the scientists" were unfounded.

Kushner then called in one of his administrative assistants for input. She said it would be a "bad idea." It was, she instructed me, not smart to "upset" Dr. Birx. So the roundtable was nixed.

Finally, I pushed back hard. "Absolutely not," I said, steaming. "Some of these guys are already in flight to DC. I insist the meeting occur. It's outrageous. I won't cancel it. I cannot do that now." I actually thought about quitting on the spot.

Kushner remained calm, even though I didn't. He thought carefully for a moment, then said, "OK, but there will be no press event, no discussion, just a 5-minute hello, a meet-and-greet in the Oval Office." I was grateful that Kushner was sympathetic to all that had already gone into this and was flexible enough to reconsider. Even though it seemed like a disappointment, I had no choice but to accept. I was consoled knowing we would all still meet with the vice president the following day.

* * * * *

On August 26, Drs. Bhattacharya, Kulldorff, Ladapo, and Meissner passed through White House security and were escorted to COVID testing in the EEOB. I was jubilant. I would no longer be alone howling in the wind. Additional experts would now be making the same case I had been putting forward for weeks. Still, because of the bizarre and frustrating hurdles leading up to this day, part of me wasn't confident we'd pull this thing off.

Once everyone was tested, we grabbed a bite from the EEOB cafeteria and caught up in my office. I downloaded the saga, explaining to them how this whole thing almost fell apart one day earlier. We then walked over to the West Wing. I introduced the group to John Rader and Derek Lyons, and we all headed upstairs for our Oval Office meeting.

The group was in awe of the classically adorned and historic Roosevelt Room. And we sat there for almost an hour. I wanted us to be there far in advance of the meeting. During that time, I oriented everyone again to what I anticipated would occur. I warned them it would be extremely short. I would introduce them to the president, and then I assumed the president would take control, say "hello," and that would probably be it. I assured the group that this trip was worthwhile. The substantive meeting would occur tomorrow, with the vice president, the head of the Task Force.

A staffer entered the Roosevelt Room to escort us to the Oval Office. As we crossed the hallway, I told everyone to leave their phones in the anteroom and reminded them: "Be concise, be direct, and answer questions with the truth. That's why you're here."

As we entered, the president gestured for us to approach the *Resolute* Desk, with his usual smile and friendly welcome. We sat in a semicircle of chairs, now numbering five. I handed the bios of our guests to the president and began the introductions. In my head, I visualized the five-minute timer starting to tick down. Without wasting any time, I went around the room.

"Mr. President, I will quickly introduce everyone, if that's OK." The president nodded, hands folded on the desk, signaling with a nod to proceed.

With each introduction, the president nodded, smiled, and said, "Thank you. Thank you for coming." Afterward, he said, "Thank you, Scott, for this. I really appreciate it." Then, looking from visitor to visitor, then around the room at his advisors both on the periphery and behind us on the sofas, he exclaimed, "We have five geniuses here!"

The president was fired up, and I was relieved to see we had done the right thing. I did not want those at the highest levels in the White House to think I was wasting the time of the commander in chief.

What followed was completely unexpected but, in retrospect, classic Trump. He eagerly commandeered the meeting. This was not going to be a quick "hello."

The president began by diving into the important issues of the pandemic, posing questions to each doctor and listening intently to their responses.

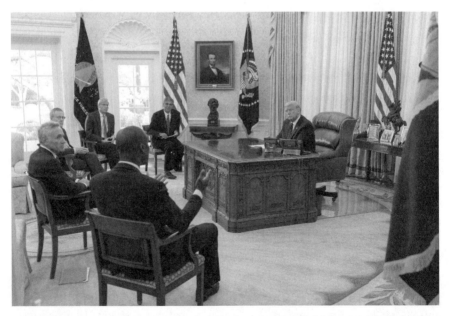

In our secret meeting with expert physicians and scientists in the Oval Office, President Trump listened intently to Dr. Joe Ladapo. I looked on next to Dr. Ladapo, while to my left, Drs. Cody Meissner, Martin Kulldorff, and Jay Bhattacharya (far side) also listened. (*Credit: Official White House photographers*)

He asked, for example, whether he did the right thing with the initial shutdown—and proceeded to opine. He asked about the trends in the United States and how our country compared to others. He asked about what was happening in Asia. He asked whether the schools should open. What about the lockdowns? Where is this all headed? When will this end? Who should be tested? What's the point of testing healthy young people? He relayed his favorite nonquestion about what would likely happen if his son Barron contracted COVID: "He would probably have the sniffles and then feel fine, right?"

On every topic that came up during the meeting, he turned to me, asking for comments and posing additional questions. This was the president's standard behavior, and it was apparent whenever I was in one of the chairs in the Oval Office. He would frequently turn to me and comment, even when the discussion was totally unrelated to health care, sometimes just to joke or make an aside. At a separate meeting, the president started discussing taxes with Treasury Secretary Steven Mnuchin, and I also happened to be in the room. He broke off conversation, laughing, and said, "Scott, I bet you wish you were back at Stanford right now, don't you?!"

I checked my watch. We had been in the Oval Office for more than half an hour! Right then, I felt a tap on my shoulder. I think it was Hicks who handed me a handwritten note card: "5 minutes." I nodded affirmatively, but there was no way I was going to interrupt the president. Then he stood up and boomed, "Get the cameras in here!" The White House photographer snapped away. Still today, I look at the photos and shake my head at the stupid political decision to hide the event from the public. He then had a White House photographer come in with a video camera.

"Scott, why don't you discuss what is going on?" President Trump instructed.

Meadows was standing there, impatiently, since this was now a forty-five-minute intrusion into a jam-packed schedule. But of course, the president was in charge. I began speaking to a camera, giving several minutes of off-the-cuff remarks about the meeting, the participants, and the issues.

I laughed inside at all the handwringing that had occurred trying to block an event that the president was obviously thrilled to hold. Perhaps I would also win out on getting some public visibility for this discussion? I couldn't help but remember my lack of respect for "political strategists," something I acquired while advising Rudy Giuliani on health care during the 2008 presidential campaign. The people Giuliani had brought on board were an abject failure, squandering his lead and destroying his momentum.

Finally, Meadows stepped forward and said, "Mr. President, we really need to move on." As he often did with guests, the president invited each of the invited doctors to pose for a photo with him behind the *Resolute* Desk. We also took a group photo. Jay quickly grabbed a chart that he made of CDC trends—one that the president had shown during a recent press briefing—and the president autographed it at his desk.

Mission accomplished. We left the Oval Office.

*   *   *   *   *

We were all set to continue the conversation the following day with Vice President Pence. This was going to be highly impactful, I told everyone, because the VP ran the Task Force meetings. After this, he would be armed with data and knowledge that no one but me ever brought up.

The meeting was set for Thursday, August 27 in the Roosevelt Room. I reminded everyone beforehand that time was very tight, so please be concise and direct if asked a question. My dealings with the VP had always been very positive, and I reassured everyone that he was highly interested in hearing the facts. The schools would certainly be one of the topics discussed. As everyone waited in the Roosevelt Room, I walked over toward the VP's West Wing office; together, we walked back into the conference room, where all seats had been assigned with name placards.

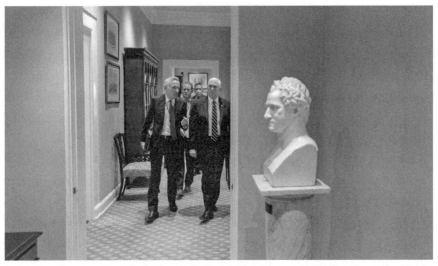

Approacing the meeting with visiting medical scientists, I prepped Vice President Pence in the hallway upstairs in the West Wing, carrying my folder full of journal articles. *(Credit: Official White House photographers)*

After the VP opened with pleasantries, I introduced everyone. He asked some pointed questions, and each of us briefed him on schools, the risk to children, the role of testing, and other key issues. Pence was eager to learn and listened intently.

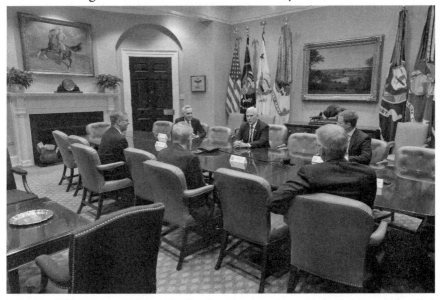

In the West Wing's Roosevelt Room, Vice President Pence ran the meeting with the panel of medical scientists. Across from VP Pence sat Professors Bhattacharya (smiling), Meissner, and Kulldorff (left to right), while I sat on the same side as the vice president and his staff member. *(Credit: Official White House photographers)*

Following the half-hour meeting, he asked for a summary document explaining the literature on schools and children, saying, "I am an avid reader, I like to go through the data and understand it." That was excellent, I thought, because the data was clear. I replied that I would compile it with Jay Bhattacharya. The group of us then left and headed to my EEOB office, where I had prepared some souvenir bags for the experts to take home for their children.

Once again, the communications team had been prepped with the stellar bios of the visitors, and we had discussed potential media outreach in detail. However, no publicity was permitted documenting the visit of the group of expert doctors and scientists with the VP. No press release, no photos to the media, no press briefing, no media interaction. And once again, I was stunned by the lack of any desire to reassure the public that the president and VP were engaged with top national experts. In my mind, it was extremely positive that our nation's leaders were seeking this kind of qualified input. Who in their right minds would not agree with that approach? Shouldn't the false claim that this president, this vice president, did not "listen to the science" be rebutted?

Instead, the decision was quite the opposite. The communications side and the political team advising the White House lived in fear of the reaction from a relentlessly hostile media. They thought only of the downside, that it would show disharmony among the Task Force. They were held hostage by the potential reaction in the press from Fauci and Birx. It did not matter to the internal political advisors that Birx had turned down the invitation to attend the Oval Office meeting. No one seemed to agree that it was a positive thing to project an administration seeking expert advice. Instead I heard, over and over again, from Mark Meadows and Marc Short: "We don't want to rock the boat, Scott." Yes, I know, we are only a couple of months from the election.

Two key documents arose out of these meetings. First, I asked Jay to send me an updated version of a document for the VP about pediatric transmission of the virus that he had shared with me when we were both helping in a discussion about schools opening. Second, Jay and Martin quickly coauthored an op-ed for the *Wall Street Journal*, published on September 3, entitled "The Case Against Covid Tests for the Young and Healthy," which discussed why schools should be reopened; explained the flaws in the principle of testing young, healthy people; and emphatically endorsed the new but controversial CDC testing guidance.

I felt it was urgent that the VP see the scientific evidence on schools right away, because I had spoken about the data at a recent Task Force meeting. In addition, I made sure Jay included my findings behind why cases surged in Israel when schools reopened back in May. The Israeli experience had been serving as a key data point to justify the need to keep schools closed. The problem was, the assertion that opening schools had caused cases to surge was totally wrong.

Soon after arriving in Washington, I had asked one of my best outside analysts to examine the Israeli social mobility data, specifically from the weeks before their schools opened. That data had already been archived off the Google tracking website, but he persevered and dug it up. It had been claimed in the media that Israel had been locked down, generally isolated, until schools reopened, after which cases surged. But that was false. For more than three weeks leading up to the reopening, social mingling and mobility had dramatically increased—in nearly every examined part of society and every examined region. Across the board, Israel had begun to mingle, moving around 80 percent or more back to their normal baseline seen without any restrictions at all. From that research, the conclusion that it was May's school reopening that caused cases to surge was patently invalid—another instance of what I called "sloppy thinking from smart people."

The vice president received my analysis a few days after our meeting, and Bhattacharya and Kulldorff included it in their op-ed on testing asymptomatic young people. Finally, many months later, on January 18, 2021, my analysis was validated in *Clinical Infectious Diseases*, an official publication of the Infectious Diseases Society of America, in a study out of Israel that concluded, "School reopening on May 2020 did not have a major effect on SARS-CoV-2 resurgence in Israel during June-July. Rather, the easing of restrictions on large-scale gatherings was primarily responsible for this resurgence, and the increased hospitalizations and mortality." Nevertheless, the original erroneous and harmful conclusion was never corrected by the experts who claimed the opposite, and it was never corrected by the media, even today.

CHAPTER 14
Rebutting the Science Deniers

Regardless of the absurdity of the personal attacks, I was really worried that the media attack on me was undermining the validity of my message. That was a huge problem, even though the president, most of the inner circle of his advisors, and a contingent of those leading the agencies on the Task Force agreed with my logic of focusing protection on the high-risk population while opening schools and society. To me, no matter how frustrating the abysmal lack of scientific knowledge on the part of the Task Force doctors and their incomprehensible disregard for the harms of the lockdowns, the public's understanding was what would change the momentum. That meant I could not go it alone.

I called Martin Kulldorff who had already written a letter to the heavily politicized Stanford student newspaper defending me, after a group of medical school faculty wrote their scurrilous, unhinged rebuke. Of course, the professors had refused his challenge to debate the issue, but that was understandable, since the signatories did not include Stanford's most knowledgeable infectious disease epidemiologists, all of whom supported me.

I suggested to Martin that we hold a highly visible panel discussion in front of the Washington media to show the world that experts in epidemiology and infectious disease agreed with the strategy I was advocating. I was also highly interested in adding Oxford's Sunetra Gupta, who had been highly vocal in supporting the same targeted protection of the known vulnerable while opening schools and society. She was one of the first to cast doubt on the initial models and was stunned at how those models were taken as accurate for basing unprecedented, draconian lockdowns. She was also vocal about the lack of sense underlying mass testing to define cases in this pandemic and shocked at the systemic disregard of fundamental immunology and infectious disease knowledge. Moreover, she too had been pilloried in the media back in the UK. Somehow, her official title of "theoretical epidemiologist" disqualified her from having an opinion, even though she was one of the world's leading authorities on the epidemiology and immunology of infectious diseases, including having developed a clinical influenza vaccine that might obviate the need for a new flu vaccine every year.

I asked Martin if he knew Sunetra. Fortunately, he had already been arranging a distance-based interview that he hoped would include her, while he and Jay were going to be in Massachusetts. It was perfect timing.

Martin told Sunetra that I had an idea to hold a live panel discussion in Washington and that I would like her to attend. He noted that I had a Plan A, B, and C, but it was still a work in progress. To get the most media coverage, I first hoped to bring everyone in to meet the president, but later that was taken off the table—not just from political sensitivities of everyone, but I didn't want this to be politicized and thereby delegitimized.

Sunetra agreed to fly to Washington, if she could get around travel restrictions, of course. I immediately began asking around the West Wing how to arrange her travel clearance. Meanwhile Martin came up with a way to fund her trip, with help from a small economic institute in Massachusetts called the American Institute of Economic Research. Martin and Jay were already organizing their idea of a video interview.

Simultaneously, I was scrambling to figure out how to make sure this event received prominent coverage by the media. I knew that if I was associated with the panel, it would be portrayed as political, so I insisted to Martin that I could not be part of a public panel. The media was hostile to any opinion contrary to the accepted narrative; even some of those who had published my op-eds and had tremendous success in attracting viewers were now reluctant, sadly cowering to the anti-Trump pressure.

Meanwhile, after several conversations with his close advisors, Secretary Azar agreed to host an informal meeting with Kulldorff, Bhattacharya, Gupta, and me. I was thrilled but still anxious. I was reminded that it needed to be run by Kushner or someone high level in the White House. I really did not want to do that, remembering the fiasco of a month earlier and their misguided fear of alienating Birx before the election. I eventually mentioned it to Kushner, although in a casual way, and it was fine—it wasn't in the White House, so that gave it some distance, I assumed. I gave the word to HHS that it was acceptable to move forward.

I spoke with Azar's staff about arranging media coverage, including a press release—that was all set, they assured me. The meeting would occur at HHS. "Awesome," I thought. "That is pretty high profile."

On the afternoon before her flight, Sunetra still had no official approval to fly to the US. At the last minute, I frantically succeeded in getting DHS to arrange her security clearance. I emailed her on October 1 that it was set. I was so relieved, actually amazed that this was accomplished, given all the hurdles.

My relief didn't last long. That same day, the president tested positive for COVID and was admitted to Walter Reed Hospital. The media frenzy was palpable, as was the fear inside the West Wing, and of course the communications team was freaking out. The insanity of it all was surreal. It was not the main issue at this point, but clearly there was no chance of getting media attention at our planned live event. I was informed by someone still trying to organize it that everyone in the media was going to be camped out at the hospital. The tumult about the president, though, was not going to stop this meeting from occurring, I reassured myself.

I arrived thirty minutes early in the lobby of the Humphreys Building. When Jay, Martin, and Sunetra walked in, I was literally overjoyed. I also thought, naively again, that this would finally destroy the vicious media distortions about me purveying "pseudoscience" and the nonstop accusations that the president "didn't listen to the science." I knew I could never thank them enough, especially Sunetra, for putting themselves in the firing line.

We took the elevators up after the temperature checks in the lobby and were escorted into one of the HHS conference rooms. Our name tags were dutifully spaced around the large table. We took our photos—in the back of my mind, I did not trust that this would ever become visible any other way.

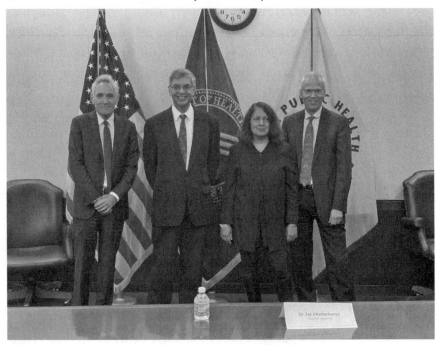

I stood proudly in the HHS conference room with Stanford's Jay Bhattacharya, Oxford's Sunetra Gupta, and Harvard's Martin Kulldorff as we awaited our meeting with Secretary Alex Azar. (*Credit: Personal photograph*)

In walked the Secretary Azar, his highly capable advisor Paul Mango, and one or two other staff. Azar asked numerous questions, and we all spoke freely. The key topics were covered—risks to children, the idea of protecting the high-risk groups instead of locking down and isolating everyone, the harms of school closures, the limited utility of masks, the impact of lockdowns on working class and poor families. We spoke about the concept of herd immunity and how that had become totally distorted, as if it were not a biological principle. No one advocated allowing the infection to spread without mitigation, and we each spoke of how to further increase protection. Instead of focusing on my own views, I tried to ensure that the secretary heard directly from the panel. My role was mainly to see that all the important topics were brought up. Several official photos were then taken to document and, I thought, publicize the event. In short, it was a smashing success. I couldn't wait to see the media coverage once the photos and the formal press release announced the proceedings.

We all exited the room and grabbed lunch together in the HHS cafeteria. Smiles were everywhere. I immediately tried to set up some interviews while still inside the building. Martin needed to fly back to his family that afternoon, but Jay and Sunetra would join me for a celebratory dinner that night at my hotel. The BBC agreed to interview the trio, with Martin via distance (I said I would not participate, because I did not want to detract by my radioactive association with the administration). Laura Ingraham of Fox News was interested in a TV spot that night. I also informed *The Hill* and some other media outlets about the meeting.

At dinner, we toasted our success. We discussed the lockdowns, the media distortions, the shocking lack of critical thinking by government leaders and scientists throughout the world. We talked about the vicious hostility, not just from the media but from our academic colleagues in the US and UK. In the middle of dinner, I suddenly remembered the BBC interview. I called them; they now said they had changed their minds, but had not even told me. I bluntly said it was unprofessional and asked what was going on. After months of featuring experts claiming the need for lockdowns without any other view in sight, the BBC now said they would only interview Sunetra, Martin, and Jay if experts on "the other side of the argument" were also included. I told them they were only interested in censoring the debate; they clearly never had insisted on that for months as they interviewed pro-lockdown advocates. All of us were stunned.

Then the time came for the Laura Ingraham interview, with Jay and Sunetra sitting alongside each other while Martin dialed in from Boston. I had another glass of wine and waited at our table.

Our celebration did not last long. The lies and distortions came immediately. *The Hill* headlined their report, "Trump health official meets with doctors pushing herd immunity"—published as news, not opinion—even after speaking directly to both me and

Bhattacharya that same day. In it, the author claimed we advised "allowing the virus to spread uncontrollably." We both immediately wrote the reporter directly, emphasizing that we never pushed any such strategy, that we absolutely did not advocate that. She disregarded our direct, written words, and instead *The Hill* disgracefully stuck to their distortion. *Politico* also put forth their straw-man accusation: "Trump advisers consult scientists pushing disputed herd immunity strategy," adding the doomsday threat that "experts say that seeking widespread immunity in the manner the scientists prescribe could result in the deaths of hundreds of thousands or even millions more U.S. residents." Even *Forbes* repeated the distortion: "The Trump Administration Goes All In on Herd Immunity"; and the usual CNN-*Washington Post*-*New York Times* echo chamber reverberated loudly throughout the world. It was a full-blown war on truth.

Yet again, instead of assuring the public that their president and his administration were listening to world renowned experts, there was almost no publicity from the administration and none from the White House that the event had occurred. No press release. No media. No release of any official photos. In the end, I was extremely grateful to see the tweet or two sent out from Secretary Azar's team, something that I had to directly push for until they were finally released.

CHAPTER 15
POTUS Gets COVID

Early Friday morning, October 2, in the midst of organizing details about the visit from the trio of epidemiologists to Washington, I was told the president had tested positive for COVID and was headed to Walter Reed for care. The president himself broke the news in his customary way—via Twitter. Soon thereafter, he was taken to the hospital.

My first thought was the president's health. I was concerned but calm, reassured first and foremost that he was going to the hospital. At the same time, I had confidence in the outcome, because the president was relatively healthy—sure, overweight and older, but there was no one I had ever encountered with more energy, more vigor, at that age. I was absolutely certain that he would not want to be hospitalized—that was totally opposite to his personality—but I also felt strongly that it would be reckless to do anything but ensure the president of the United States was in a highly monitored hospital setting with immediate access to all necessary treatment.

The news coverage was immediately on fire, understandably. Speculation was rampant. And as expected from a reckless, hyperbolic press, that speculation was sensationalistic to the max, even though it was pure hearsay, based on almost nothing factual. Kayleigh, as always, was spot on, reassuring the press that "out of an abundance of caution" he had been taken to the hospital. In contrast, the communications team immediately stumbled, making unforced errors in interviews, even commenting unnecessarily on "vital signs" as if they had any perspective about that, and further implying the situation was very precarious. To me, admittedly a total neophyte about public relations, that was a huge blunder, almost inexplicable. "OK," I thought, "whatever. Not my job."

Not unexpectedly, I was also contacted by the press. I explained that I had no special information about the president's condition and, even if I did, there was zero chance I would reveal it. That said, I thought it would have been a mistake if absolutely nothing at all was said—that might imply something was being covered up, which was not the case. That would invoke unnecessary fear, the last thing the American public needed. I therefore gave a very simple statement to the reporter: the president was a healthy, vigorous man, and even though he was a senior citizen, we expected him to do well and return to work.

This should not have been controversial. Why wouldn't I remain calm, given the data on the virus? Shouldn't the entire White House remain composed? The American public deserved sensible, calmly delivered information. My statement was a very generic, levelheaded communication, fully consistent with the extensive body of data on how well the overwhelming majority of people do with COVID, other than those who are high-risk and frail. And absolutely no objective person who ever spent any time with President Trump would conclude that he was not a very vigorous, energetic man—the opposite of frail. There was literally nothing problematic about my short statement—I said nothing at all about his condition, and never even implied I knew those details.

Yet, the communications team overreacted almost immediately. I was told to stop all interviews, period. I wasn't the only one who was muzzled—but I was personally informed that all interviews set up for that day would be cancelled until further notice. That was "an ORDER" directly from the chief of staff, according to the people on the team. That was not a problem for me at all, but I wasn't the only one who disagreed. Several others inside the West Wing kept telling me to talk with reporters, given that I was the only clinically experienced doctor on the entire team outside his physicians, that I was capable of speaking on COVID, and that I was specifically the president's advisor on the subject. But I declined all interviews, especially since I had no interest in speaking with the press anyway. Unfortunately, that left even more speculation and misinformation to spread. Ironically, I found out the next morning that the president also disagreed with that "stand down" approach to the media—he was angry about that decision.

The following morning, I telephoned the hospital, standing anxiously beside the desk in my hotel room. I was put through to the President in his hospital room.

"Hi, Scott!" he began.

"Hello, Mr. President, how do you feel?"

"I feel great! I want to get the hell outta here!" he boomed.

I laughed, thinking, "Of course!" Just as I expected, he was like a caged animal, outside his element, isolated from the public, raring to return to work.

He continued, telling me he had a group of expert doctors from all over the country at his side, taking great care of him. He sounded very upbeat, already noticeably anxious to come back to the White House. He asked me what I thought about his team of doctors, saying who they were and what institutions they were from. I reassured him that his team was of course outstanding, that I had every confidence in his doctors, and that he should trust them completely. He asked what I thought about the medications he was on. I assured him that Dr. Conley and the entire team were certainly on top of all the latest available drugs. I had great confidence in his care, and so should he.

In this situation, where a patient is rightfully concerned about their health, there is nothing more important for a trusted physician to do than reassure the patient. I have seen how overwhelming it is for a patient to be surrounded by a cadre of doctors, and that's especially true for all "VIP patients" whom I have consulted on during my career. I understood that the president was asking just like any ordinary patient would—he might have been the president, but he was still a human being. He also trusted, first and foremost, that I would always tell him the truth.

I then gave the president my update about what I saw in the White House. From the first awareness of his positive test, panic had emerged in the West Wing. I mentioned that everyone was scurrying around, suddenly wearing masks everywhere, frantically setting new rules about behavior, even contemplating issuing new statements about mandates. When I first walked upstairs in the West Wing on hearing about the president's positive test, Kushner and everyone else were wearing masks, whereas the day before almost no one did. Before I could say a word, Kushner turned to me and said, "I know, this is silly, right?" pointing to his new mask. I smiled and said nothing; nothing needed to be said.

Somehow, most people in the White House took this one infection as requiring a sudden change in policies that had been in place for months. Not everyone, though. Johnny McEntee made the commonsense deduction before anyone else the next morning: "Since the only point of our daily testing was to protect the boss," he observed, "then I guess we should be finished with testing, right?" He laughed as we awaited our tests with Kayleigh in the EEOB that weekend. Like most irrational behavior during the pandemic, virtually everyone in the West Wing now began getting tested, regardless of whether they had been anywhere near the president.

On the same call that Saturday morning, President Trump abruptly instructed, "Tell everyone there, call Jason, no new Tweet, tell Kayleigh, nothing has changed. No mask mandate, it's still 'masks only if you cannot socially distance' like always. No masks required in West Wing, there is nothing different, absolutely nothing." Then he exclaimed with irritation in his voice, "Where the hell is everyone? Where are the interviews, I see no one on TV!?" Dr. Fauci kept on interviewing, of course, positing the ever-present, potentially negative turn of events that never happened. Nothing would stop that, and no one ever tried. I told the president that I didn't know about others, but I was shut down, being told unequivocally that Meadows had said absolutely no interviews. The president was frustrated, angry; he didn't know why that would be the case. I told him to rest up, not realizing he was already figuring out his next move.

Sitting at my table having breakfast in the lobby of the Trump Hotel, I found it impossible to avoid watching the breathless reporting on the four large-screen TVs. The next day, it did not shock me one bit to see the president waving to his supporters from the back of the limo circling the hospital. Needless to say, no one in the West Wing could have been surprised. Everyone knew he was irrepressible, full of energy, and absolutely unaccepting about being confined inside a hospital room when he already felt "great!"

Just as expectedly, the outpouring of hand-wringing, disapproval, and consternation from all the "experts" filled the cable news networks and the press. "How outrageous Trump is!" they shouted. As usual, every reporter and talking head was suddenly an expert, apoplectic at every action by this president. I already knew the president was doing well; indeed, I fully expected him to be released within a couple of days, but he would likely stay hospitalized for now since he was being given IV medication. At this point, the media frenzy was full blown, and although totally expected, it made this whole episode surreal.

CHAPTER 16
The Election Approaches

Task Force meetings became somewhat erratic in October due to the VP's campaign schedule, and that made it easier for me to skip a couple of them. However, I continued to work hard trying to improve the protection of high-risk Americans.

For those weeks, CMS Administrator Seema Verma and I communicated on an almost daily basis to ramp up protection of the elderly. Every day, I would stay on top of the infection activity in every state through COVID patients coming to the emergency rooms. From that monitoring, I would alert Seema. She would then organize calls or other means to notify the relevant state nursing home agencies to immediately increase the staff testing. The goal was to interrupt the introduction of infections into their region's nursing homes. Seema and I were particularly concerned that issuing guidelines might not be enough, so she repeatedly alerted nursing homes and instituted tracking protocols for accountability. Liaisons with hospitals to improve infection control in nursing homes were another piece of the solution.

For seniors living outside nursing homes, I would also meet with Brad Smith of domestic policy and Seema to figure out ways to send more point-of-care tests, more PPE, and other resources to visiting nursing agencies and nonresidential community centers frequented by seniors. I also pushed for the use of an existing alert system to community Medicare recipients who were at particular risk so they, too, would be aware of surging infection activity in their communities. That would heighten their awareness to enforce stricter distancing and other mitigation measures at home. These were very productive collaborations.

As October came to a close, the upcoming election became the topic of almost every casual discussion around the White House. The president was on the campaign trail in full force, visibly energized by the crowds. His own enjoyment of the interaction with the public translated into some overly optimistic chatter throughout the EEOB and West Wing but mainly by people who knew nothing beyond cable news reports and their own gut feelings.

And then, just days before the voting, I received a series of extraordinary phone calls from different members of the Task Force.

The first came from Dr. Brett Giroir, the director of the testing program, while I sat at my desk reading new journal publications. He began by asking, "Are you still in Washington?" Since my main contact with him had been at the Task Force meetings, my absence had been noticeable. I answered, "Absolutely, yes, working hard, trying to get things done rather than go to meetings. I decided to skip the Task Force the last couple of meetings, though. It was a waste of time for me; no one cared about the data," I bluntly said. At this point, there was no reason to be diplomatic.

Giroir then shocked me. Out of nowhere, he declared, "It looks like the president is going to win. We really need to reconfigure the Task Force. This is the time to do it. We absolutely need to get rid of Birx."

I replied with a noncommittal, "Really?"

Giroir went on. "She cannot work with anyone. She just goes full speed ahead without consulting anyone. She's extremely difficult, she flies off the handle at any criticism, and she doesn't understand the data. The president needs to get rid of her."

I was flabbergasted, but I began to laugh. After all this time, Giroir, the picture of loyalty, was trying to put a knife into Birx's back. I wasn't sure if he was being sincere or just trying to save his own position, but I took him at his word. I assumed that Giroir must have been convinced that if the president was reelected, then I would stay on and I would apparently hold some influence. His assumption was incorrect. I had already decided to leave, no matter what. But there was no reason to confide this to him.

I answered, "Thanks for the insights; let's see what happens in the election."

The next day, I was walking under the awning at the entrance to the West Wing when my phone rang. Seema Verma grumbled to me in a friendly way how she was "left alone" at the most recent Task Force meeting, because I had skipped it. This basically stranded her and the other few willing to question what was said. Seema laughingly related that she was frantically looking around as the usual outlandish nonsense was being put forth, knowing that I would have been the one to push back.

Then she got to the point. "Scott, we need to get rid of Birx. She is a disaster! She keeps saying the same things over and over; she's incredibly insecure; she doesn't understand what's going on. We need to eliminate her moving forward."

Standing in the foyer of the West Wing, I shook my head and laughed inside. I already knew that Seema was often skeptical of the misinformation spouted by Fauci and Birx, so it didn't completely shock me. Unlike Giroir, though, Seema did not directly mention the upcoming election in the call. That did not hide the obvious—she thought the momentum of the election was shifting, so the president might actually be reelected. If President Trump was reelected, she concluded that he would finally disband what had become a completely dysfunctional Task Force. Of course, Seema also knew what I thought about Birx. We continued the call for more than twenty minutes, commiserated about various things that had transpired over the previous few months, and ended by saying, "Well, let's wait and see what happens."

* * * * *

By October, the beginning of Birx's impulse to run from accountability was implied in one very important but calculating way: it seemed to me that she suddenly understood the word "lockdown" was a negative. Apparently, after I had repeatedly explained in the media that lockdowns were killing people, sacrificing our children, and destroying lower-income families, I guessed that she perceived that Kushner and the others at the COVID Huddles might have been partly swayed. It may also have occurred to her, as it had to Giroir and Seema Verma, that the president might win reelection and that their very public disagreement over policy would ultimately be resolved in his favor.

As I was explaining the harms of the policies yet again at another painful COVID Huddle, Birx interrupted me from across the table. She looked at me, then at the others around the room, shaking her head, and insisted, "No one on the Task Force is for lockdowns; none of the doctors are!"

I immediately put forth a series of questions, directly to her.

"Are you for testing healthy, asymptomatic people?"

She answered, "Yes."

"What will you do with that information?"

"Quarantine them for fourteen days," she answered matter-of-factly.

I asked if schools should be closed if kids tested positive.

"Yes."

"And are you for closing bars and restaurants and restricting other businesses?"

"Yes!" she adamantly declared.

Thoroughly exasperated, I exclaimed, "That IS the definition of lockdowns! Simply saying, 'I'm against lockdowns,' and then advising policies that result in lockdowns is being FOR lockdowns!"

*　*　*　*　*

One of the routine agenda items at the COVID Huddle was an update on the vaccine progress. At one Huddle, a few weeks before the election, the decision was made to announce the successful development of the vaccine as soon as the data was known and revealed. Everyone had already witnessed several interviews in which officials inside and outside the administration cast doubt on the possibility that a vaccine could be developed before year's end. Those were contrary to the facts, but such claims were everywhere, no doubt politically motivated. And clearly, the Emergency Use Authorization was not going to happen before November 3. Why not? Because Stephen Hahn and the FDA unexpectedly introduced an extra delay, a requirement of sixty days between half the test subjects receiving the dose and a safety assessment of the mRNA vaccines in trials.

I was informed by a highly experienced vaccine expert who had worked with the FDA and CDC for years that this exceeded the standard forty-two days typically needed to assess safety issues. No one can know with certainty the motivation of adding extra delays, but given that the world was paralyzed by the pandemic, it certainly smelled of politics. Delaying a lifesaving vaccine for political concerns seems almost inconceivable, but we had already seen inexcusable, blatantly political comments from our leading politicians that likely cost lives. I do not suspect any illicit motivation, but Americans might be interested to learn that on June 22, 2021, Hahn was hired by Flagship Pioneering Co.—the venture capital firm that launched the Moderna mRNA vaccine and that still owns a significant stake in the company.

Even though the FDA seemed to have delayed the possibility of revealing successful clinical trial data until after the vote, those in the Roosevelt Room knew that the efficacy data would be ready beforehand. Clearly, no one could see the efficacy data until it was looked at by the outside expert committee, the Data and Safety Management Board, but that first look was on schedule to occur before the election. Everyone also understood that showing vaccine success alone would be exciting news, even if the final assessment came later, and would likely provide a boost to the president's chances.

Regardless of what the clinical trial would show, the bold strategic idea behind Operation Warp Speed was the decision to remove most of the financial risk from the companies by buying the doses up-front, while simultaneously organizing the logistics of production and delivery in advance. Therefore the estimated numbers of doses and deliveries were reviewed at the COVID Huddles. As I had done a number of times for the media, I mentioned the numbers and timing estimates at the COVID Huddle, which I had just gone over with Paul Mango of HHS.

To my great surprise, Dr. Birx protested the numbers as the meeting closed. She repeatedly said, "No, that's not true; we will not have the vaccine that quickly, and we will not have anywhere near those numbers; we cannot say that." I was incredulous. I got up and gestured to Paul, who was standing in the periphery of the Roosevelt Room. By then, people were standing around the table, some exiting. I replied, "Wait a second, Paul and I were just looking at the numbers; those numbers are exactly what the agreements say!" But Birx kept denouncing the estimates, shaking her head.

I wondered, "Why in the world would she dispute numbers right out of the original documents?" Downplaying the near-term availability of the vaccine would prevent positive information from coming out before the election, whether politics was the motivation or not.

* * * * *

Days later, as everyone in the West Wing anticipated the upcoming reveal of the clinical trial data, a new delay appeared. The enrollment numbers were known, but it was not certain how many cases of COVID had been experienced by the trial subjects. The determination of success or failure rested on the statistical analysis of infections in the placebo group compared to the vaccinated group.

Then Pfizer's leadership abruptly announced that their scheduled look at the first thirty-two cases of COVID, highly likely from all estimates to occur in October, was no longer the plan. According to *Stat News*, William Gruber, Pfizer's senior vice president of vaccine clinical research and development, said they had decided not to conduct the thirty-two-case analysis. Instead, they would conduct it later, after sixty-two cases of COVID had arisen.

As it turned out, there had already been ninety-four cases of COVID in the trial (triple the necessary thirty-two for statistical significance). This means that if Pfizer had held to their original plan, the data would have been available in October, as its CEO, Albert Bourla, initially predicted. That was also the prediction of HHS, one that the president and I separately echoed at the press briefings and in the media.

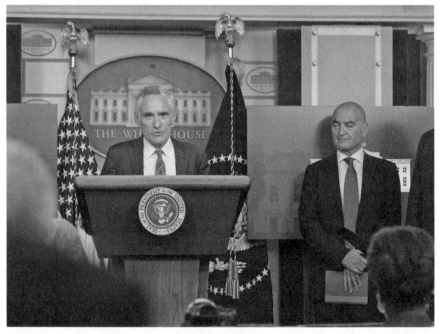

Answering press questions about the vaccine from the podium while Moncef Slaoui, the leader of the OWS vaccine development, and President Trump looked on. (*Credit: Official White House photographers*)

I still do not know why the decision was made to delay looking at the data until after the election.

CHAPTER 17
The Florida Success Story

For several months before coming to Washington, I had already been speaking with Governor Ron DeSantis about the pandemic in Florida. Florida was always in particular danger from this virus, because of its unique demographics. It has an especially vulnerable population, since more than 4.4 million seniors live there. By percentage, Florida ranks the second highest of all states in residents over sixty-five years of age, and it has more than 440 certified nursing homes. The percentage of highly vulnerable groups also skewed toward minorities. Governor DeSantis was acutely aware of the risks for his constituents, so he had been discussing the situation with several outside experts, as well as Florida officials, since the early days of the pandemic.

The demographics, though, were not the real reason why Florida was exceptional. The genuine difference lay in the state's leadership. Governor DeSantis stood out among governors, because he was one of the very few who actually knew the data. And when I say he knew the data, I mean he personally sought out, critically analyzed, and truly understood every important detail about the pandemic. It was all about attention to detail, critical thinking, and a willingness to question the prevailing narrative when it did not pass the test of common sense.

It also required one more trait—the strength of personality to withstand the political heat when acting on the facts, even when the chosen path was contrary to the recommendations of the media's anointed experts and the often erratic guidelines by the CDC. It required leaders who trusted Americans, as free individuals, to manage their own lives based on proper information and guidance. South Dakota's Governor Kristi Noem also understood that—she was the single governor who did not require any businesses to close, because every business is essential to the employees and families who depend on it. Although these traits should have been expected of any responsible official, most of the nation's other governors suffered from a gross deficit of these essential characteristics.

Governor DeSantis would use most of our calls for one main purpose—to test his understanding of the data. It was almost never the case that he had a need for an answer to his questions; more typically, he would tell me his own analysis, then ask if he was correct. Without fail, he was spot-on with his analysis. That level of understanding carried far beyond the data in Florida. The governor was well aware of the current science, including new research publications, as well as trends about cases, hospitalizations, and deaths in other states and other countries. He would also bounce his ideas off me about seasonality, population susceptibility and immunity, cross-protection and T-cells versus antibody tests, masks, and other potential reasons why cases would decline.

In short, he had a solid command of virtually every aspect of the virus and the impacts of the lockdowns, the school closures, and the translation of economic devastation into lives lost. It was quite impressive. It was also a breath of fresh air. He had a far more detailed understanding of the pandemic than anyone I had encountered in the Task Force. This realization made me even more depressed about the state of things in Washington, but it also gave me hope.

During one such call in August, DeSantis asked if I would come to Florida and tour his state. This was the singular exception to all the other visits from the Task Force. Every other state visit was conducted by Dr. Birx during my time in Washington. But DeSantis and I had been talking through the data for months. He fully understood the failures, the destructive impact, and the frank lack of logic of the Birx-Fauci lockdowns.

Two key aspects of his management of the pandemic were perfect for me to highlight in Florida. To protect Floridians, the governor had enacted the targeted protection of the elderly I had spoken about. For instance, he set up two dozen "COVID-only" facilities for residents who tested positive and forbade hospital discharges to nursing homes. That prevented the reintroduction of the virus back into nursing homes—something several other governors failed to do, thereby tragically killing thousands of elderly people. DeSantis had further prioritized protective equipment and more frequent testing of nursing home residents and staff. He also admitted his earlier mistake of shutting down elective medical procedures.

In addition to his focus on protecting the elderly, the governor wanted us to highlight school openings and visit some of his state's colleges. He and his education commissioner, Richard Corcoran, had issued a directive in July that all school districts should be reopened for in-person learning by the end of August. He was fully aware that the "break-outs" on university campuses highlighted by the media were misleading, because they were almost exclusively test-positive cases in healthy and asymptomatic young people with almost no risk of serious illness. At that point, tens of thousands of cases had been detected as students returned to campuses, but none had even been hospitalized. Meanwhile the Trump administration had partnered well with the State of Florida in providing economic aid, school-reopening support, medical supplies, technical assistance, and personnel.

The White House organized my trip details in concert with the governor's team in Florida. My visit commenced on August 31 at the state capitol in Tallahassee. We held a roundtable discussion and press conference that included Florida's education commissioner, a parent, and others on the progress and success of Florida's statewide school reopening. The governor outlined updated details about the virus, hospital and ICU status, and statewide testing in detail. He reviewed his focus on protecting the most vulnerable, supporting hospital capacity, and keeping schools open and society functioning.

At the press briefing, I was asked to comment on school outbreaks by the governor and to explain the new CDC testing guidelines. I emphasized the need to continue mitigation measures and testing, because "we want to protect the high-risk students, the high-risk teachers." I also noted that closing schools and colleges would be counter to the goal of protecting high-risk individuals. Schools are low-risk environments with healthier, younger populations; sending college students home would increase interaction with high-risk parents and those in their communities.

Governor DeSantis also correctly explained to the media that 90 percent of positive PCR tests were isolating people who were not contagious. That level of knowledge was not just rare for a government official; the policy implications of that fact were never even acknowledged by the other Task Force members. He also asked me specifically about asymptomatic spread. I noted it was true that asymptomatic spread occurred, but "the number one place for spread is in the home" and "from adults to children, not the other way, typically…it can happen that children spread, but that's not a common direction." I also cited data from the August 2, 2020, contact tracing study of Switzerland showing how rarely cases begin in schools. Moreover, children had been proven to have remarkably low risk from COVID all over the world, including in the US. For anyone who prioritized the education of children and young Americans, there was no scientific case for closing schools.

Toward the end, the governor brought up college football. I talked about how uniquely safe athletes were in their special environments, and DeSantis proudly announced that Florida would host the college football playoff and later the Super Bowl, noting that it should be easy to use social distancing in large, outdoor stadiums.

Lastly, some time was spent on testing. The governor noted the rarity of significant illness on campuses despite the so-called outbreaks. A reporter asked me, "Are you saying that asymptomatic spread is not a concern?" To which I replied, "No, I didn't say that." I explained, "The metric 'number of cases' is not the most important metric...it is the *impact* of those cases." I outlined new measures to heighten protection of the vulnerable, including strategically increased testing. I also called out in strong terms our nation's reluctance to reopen schools, because that policy was counter to the scientific evidence from all over the world. "We are the only country of our peer nations in the Western world who are this hysterical about opening schools," I said, thinking of the United Nations pictorial display showing virtually all nations in Western Europe and Canada had opened schools while most US schools remained closed. I further pointed out that more than two hundred thousand cases of child abuse went unreported just during the two months of spring closures, because schools were the number one agency where child abuse is noticed and reported.

Our second stop was in central Florida's Sumter County at The Villages, an impressive active retirement community. It is a collection of residential neighborhoods of over one hundred thousand people ages fifty-five and up, with recreational, leisure, and health care facilities. The Villages served as an example of how this particular illness could be successfully managed in a highly vulnerable age bracket by smartly using sensible mitigation, limiting indoor groups, but maintaining outdoor activities. The tour was followed by a visit to the University of Florida health care facility at The Villages and another roundtable discussion with several leaders of that medical complex. Another session with the press ensued.

The press conference at The Villages began with Governor DeSantis once again laying out the data—he reviewed the numbers showing Florida's trends on cases, hospitalizations, bed usage in ICUs and hospitals, and community infection levels. He reiterated his administration's focus: protecting the most vulnerable, especially the elderly in long-term care; supporting hospital capacity; and keeping schools and society functioning. Education Commissioner Corcoran noted the importance of in-person learning and described how all of Florida's school districts had been opened, and that over one million students were already attending in-person classes.

The governor then asked me to step forward. As at the earlier press conference at the state capitol, I had explained the fundamental strategy for reopening, as outlined by DeSantis: "Number one, protect the highest-risk people and save lives by doing so, and number two, making sure we don't have hospital overcrowding because, as Governor DeSantis has known throughout this, we really need to make sure medical care is given to everyone else."

I continued, "And then, of course, the third part of the strategy…is making sure that we safely open schools and the economy because we cannot sacrifice our children." I cited evidence to make a compelling, logical case to reopen. My statements were 100 percent accurate, directly based on published scientific data. I wasn't aware at the time, but the previous month, the governor's directive to open Florida schools by the end of August had also faced legal challenges from the teachers' union, falsely claiming that this would be unsafe—despite evidence from all over the world to the contrary. Again, I highlighted the tragic consequences of school closures and expressed frustration that "we seem to be the only country willing to sacrifice our children out of fear."

The questions from the press followed and immediately focused on other issues hitting the headlines, starting with the irresponsible falsehood published that very day by two *Washington Post* writers: "[Atlas] Pushes Controversial 'Herd Immunity' Strategy." That was a lie, one that logically and directly conflicted with dozens of on-the-record statements from me calling for continued and even increased mitigations when appropriate. The *Post's* intentional misrepresentation of my position, claiming that the advisor to the president of the United States was advocating for the infection to spread through the population, was intentionally provoking fear in an already terrified public. Needless to say, the false accusation was eagerly picked up and disseminated by other politically motivated outlets. It was also seized on by members of the scientific community who despised President Trump, including several Stanford faculty members who exposed themselves as either ignorant, incapable of critical analysis, or blinded by hatred of their political enemy.

I calmly explained, "The president does not have a strategy like that. I've never advocated for that strategy. So that whole discussion in the *Washington Post* was irresponsible." But the ensuing social media frenzy amplified the lie among the naive and willfully ignorant.

I took away several lessons from the trip, but none more important than what we know today. Florida had opened its schools in August 2020 and kept them open. Florida opened its theme parks, universities, and businesses, and ended its mask mandates, while the vast majority of states imposed and maintained severe societal restrictions. It must be remembered that the burden is on the states that implemented the severe restrictions on behavior—the school closures, the business shutdowns, the mask mandates, the personal curfews—to show they saved lives. Lockdown states imposed major harms, both physical and psychological harms that will last decades, whereas Florida avoided imposing those harms. If those lockdown states did not significantly outperform an open state like Florida in saving lives, then they did extraordinary harm to their citizens.

While we cannot predict the future, what are the results after one year? As of the end of spring, 2021, Florida's performance stands out as proof of the epic failure of the lockdowns recommended by Fauci and Birx, and the on-the-ground policies implemented in nearly every state of this nation. After a full year, we know the answer about Florida—the only large state that implemented a strategy of focused protection, the one large state that I personally advised during the pandemic and that rejected the Birx-Fauci strategy:

- Florida beat the national average and outperformed more than half of our states in COVID deaths per capita.

- Florida ranked first of the ten largest states in having the smallest percent excess mortality increase during the pandemic, a percent that includes deaths from the virus and the lockdown, the most valid epidemiologic statistic to compare deaths during the pandemic;

- Florida beat forty states in age-adjusted COVID mortality for the vulnerable population (aged sixty-five and over) and likewise beat approximately the same number of states for all ages. Florida had a 40 percent lower age-adjusted mortality for seniors and for all residents than the US as a whole.

- Florida far outperformed California, with its younger population, in virtually every meaningful way, an important comparison because those are similarly diverse states with a relatively similar climate but one dramatic difference—the governor of California imposed and maintained strict lockdowns, while the governor of Florida opened his state in the summer. Florida beat California on age-adjusted COVID mortality for those over sixty-five by 30 percent, on age-adjusted COVID mortality under sixty-five by 40 percent, and on percent excess mortality during the pandemic by nearly 60 percent.

- Florida avoided the extreme destruction of poor and minority populations, whereas California's policies specifically devastated them.

As I write this in summer of 2021, the latest surge in cases is now underway in certain parts of the US, including Florida and the southern US, as well as Australia, China, Japan, Mexico, and elsewhere. Just like summer of 2020, regional surges are occurring and will likely move through the country. Clearly, we again need to protect the elderly and make sure the vulnerable are vaccinated, but these latest peaks will undoubtedly decline in line with the characteristic time course. India recently surged, which caused panic and international headlines, and then the cases and deaths declined. The

UK eliminated their mandates as their cases were peaking; cases immediately declined, although the absence of media acknowledgment kept the world from knowing. Brazil surged during the southern hemisphere's 2021 winter and many lives were lost, as their vulnerable were not vaccinated and their medical system has serious challenges. That surge also created hysteria in the US and elsewhere, but now in early August, 2021, we are witnessing a dramatic decline in Brazil's cases and deaths—again, the decline is invisible in the American media.

We must also recognize this: COVID cases will continue to come and go, with a series of peaks and valleys dictated by seasonal and other variations that we must finally expect. Contagious variants will be generated that continue the spread, but in all likelihood those will be less lethal. *One thing is certain—the virus will not be eradicated by locking down society, so the appropriate focus is to limit the deaths while regaining normal life, like we do with other illnesses.* As opposed to almost all other governors, Governor DeSantis enacted the right policy almost a year ago, one that trusted Floridians with targeted protection while he opened schools and businesses in Florida. He ended the nonscientific lockdowns, mask mandates, and other nonsensical, harmful restrictions on individuals. He prioritized resources to nursing homes and implemented smart policies to increase protection of his state's extremely large population of elderly people, including prioritization of vaccines to seniors once becoming available. By doing so, he reduced the massive harms from missed medical care, avoided the enormous psychological damage to children and young adults from school closures and isolation, and stopped the tragic destruction of Floridians, especially lower-income and minority families. The lockdowns do not stop the spread of the cases, but they inflict great damage in failing to do so.

Facts matter. The governor and I were right. Period.

CHAPTER 18
Speaking the Truth to the End

The election results were in. There seemed to be an abrupt, very noticeable loss of focus, not simply an air of defeat, around the West Wing. For many in the West Wing, the political verdict was a shock, not just the end of an era.

My first thought was very different. To me, the Trump defeat meant that vaccine approvals would now come quickly. That was virtually certain, now that any possible political motivation for the delays was removed. Many people had undermined the vaccine, even the discussion about dates of the vaccine availability, all to influence the vote. In my mind, this delay, arising from a number of subtle and not-so-subtle maneuvers by those opposed to the president, represents one of the most heinous indictments of the moral vacuum I witnessed while in Washington. People apparently were so consumed by their desire to stop the reelection of this president that they did not care if people died from the delay in the vaccine approval. I was confident that the time lines I had stated about vaccine approval, production, and distribution would now be aggressively pursued—that's because those stated time lines were always verbatim from the signed contracts, regardless of the lies spewed by politicians, the false claims to the contrary by media hit pieces, and the statements emanating from others in news interviews.

For me personally, the loss by the president changed nothing. My position as advisor to the president was a 130-day limited appointment, so regardless of the winner, I was already set to leave

Washington. I had already stopped attending the Task Force meetings and the COVID Huddles by then. I had written to the VP's office that I had no time to spend teaching people who were refractory to facts. The other Task Force doctors, just days before so eager to align with me and radically reconfigure the Task Force without Dr. Birx, were stone-cold silent.

True, I had been unofficially offered several positions in a hypothetical second Trump administration. Several people in the Office of Personnel spent considerable time trying to convince me to accept a leadership position, but weeks earlier I had politely but firmly refused. I had absolutely zero interest in serving in Washington again, under any circumstances. In fact, I was eager to leave. In an effort to help, though, I had thought carefully about who would be best to fill those key positions if the president won reelection. I put forth some of the best scientists in the country as my suggestions for those posts. I regret that my recommendations for the next secretary of HHS, director of the CDC, and head of the NIH would never come to pass—the stellar people on that list, all of whom had confirmed their interest to me personally, would have brought unprecedented expertise to those positions. Hopefully, others will repair the credibility, eliminate the politicization, and elevate the academic rigor of those important agencies. Time will tell.

The next several days were eerily quiet in the West Wing. I continued to work hard trying to add resources specifically to protect high-risk Americans. I continued to strategize with others on how to deliver more tests and add protective equipment to seniors living outside residential facilities. We continued to make sure millions more tests were prioritized to Black colleges for their high-risk faculty members. We continued to ensure that nursing homes located in communities with high infection rates were alerted to test their workers more frequently. The election had no bearing on the virus; that was obvious.

As mid-November approached, I decided to ask the president to approve my plans to head home for Thanksgiving so I could be with my family in California. I called upstairs and then went into the

Oval Office. The president was sitting behind his desk and warmly said, "Hi Scott, come on in, have a seat." Ivanka Trump was standing at the front of his desk. This was the first and only time I saw her in the White House. She and I exchanged hellos as I took my usual place in the arc of four chairs, facing the president. Ivanka continued to stand at my left, just behind me, but she said nothing.

I immediately cut to the chase. "Mr. President, I plan on going back to California for Thanksgiving," and he nodded approvingly. "I am going to take a bit of time off, but I will be available there."

"Sure, that makes sense," he agreed. He then said, "You're definitely coming back; you should definitely stay, you know. I want you to come back and stay until the end; that's the best thing to do."

I was not exactly sure what I wanted to do after Thanksgiving, so I nodded but said nothing.

Then he went on. "You know, you were right. You were right about everything. You did a great job; we worked well together, had a great relationship."

I nodded and said thanks. I knew he agreed with my points about how harmful the lockdowns were, but it was reassuring to hear the president of the United States say that. I thanked him for the opportunity to help, and I said I did my best.

He repeated, "I think you should come back for the rest of the term. That's important." I replied, "I will see you soon," and we said our goodbyes. This was the shortest meeting of any time I had been in the Oval Office.

* * * * *

I finally landed back at SFO after the long flight from Dulles Airport. I had packed all my things from the hotel, because I wasn't sure when and for how long I would come back.

I came down the escalator toward the waiting area for arriving passengers. My wife was standing there. I looked at her, paused, and said, "What the hell happened?" We both laughed, but there was nothing funny about it. I felt exhausted and relieved to be back, out of the hateful freak show of Washington.

*   *   *   *   *

My break from the Washington cesspool was short-lived, even though I stayed in California. The constant flow of media hit pieces continued. The same people who wrote these lies kept trying to get my comments for their articles, as if they would present what I said with fairness or accuracy. Their game had been revealed months earlier. Even after I decided to ignore their emails laughably asking to "fact-check" their outrageous claims about me, it still amazed me how overt lies and distortions of my words were repeated over and over. Objective journalism in the United States was dead.

Added to the mix were the highly publicized criticisms by a group of uninformed, dishonest professors at Stanford, blinded by their hatred of President Trump. My appearance as an advisor to the president generated a veritable panic among them. This was more than just about science and COVID-19 policy. Every single thing I wrote and had said was completely consistent with the COVID data available to all scientists, in every detail. For months before I went to Washington, more than one hundred of my interviews and op-eds had already been read by millions, yet these writings and interviews generated no Stanford pushback. In fact, it was almost word-for-word what two of the top infectious disease epidemiologists from Stanford School of Medicine, Bhattacharya and Ioannidis, had independently stated.

What changed to provoke the attack? Let's first explore the obvious. In the 2020 presidential election, Biden won 65 percent of California votes, while Trump took 33 percent. Stanford residents voted for Biden, too—a full 94.7 percent of Stanford's exclusive 94305 zip code went to Biden; Trump received only 3.5 percent of Stanford votes, as tracked by political scientist Alvin Rabushka.

On November 19, 2020, the Stanford Faculty Senate issued a resolution condemning my work as an advisor to the president. Among their many false characterizations, they charged that I "promoted a view of COVID-19 that contradicts medical science."

In response, I issued a statement a few days later that included the following:

Unfortunately, the Stanford Faculty Senate has chosen to use its institutional voice to take sides in the debates over the complex scientific and medical questions raised by the pandemic. I fear that this precedent could further embroil the University into politics and raises the threat that the University will criticize other faculty who disagree with Stanford's institutional views on these or other issues.

By singling me out with group letters and rebukes for the exact same ideas and data put forth by two other Stanford faculty members, the political root of the censure was exposed. Virtually every scientific point I made in writing and in interviews exactly matched those of Bhattacharya and Ioannidis, including about the risk for children, spread from children, focused protection, natural immunity, masks, and the harms of lockdowns. We all correctly analyzed the science, rejected groupthink, and refused to be intimidated into silence. The difference? I alone stood on the podium, speaking to the press and the public next to President Trump.

Hoover's John Cochrane wrote what most at Stanford were afraid to even say: "What is the point of all this? There can only be one: Don't work for Republicans, don't advise them, don't deviate from the campus orthodoxy on policy issues, censor yourself from speaking unpopular opinions. And expect to be isolated, publicly shamed with vague and undocumented charges, and drummed out of the university if you do."

Although the criticisms by the Stanford professors were blatantly false and demeaned the university as a center for the free exchange of ideas, the consequences of their distortions and lies were not trivial. I was on the receiving end of a stream of vile, hate-filled threats, mostly by email but some by phone. The FBI had become involved, starting while I was still in Washington. Now that I had come back to Stanford, the university and local police forces were alerted. Among other protections, I was forced to install thousands of dollars of home security equipment. The police parked a car at my driveway 24/7. A constant security presence was visible on my street. I can only hope my Stanford colleagues and their families never experience what they recklessly instigated for mine.

* * * * *

November moved ahead very slowly, as I continued to work from home. I spent most of my time analyzing the data on the pandemic, communicating with my epidemiology colleagues about current research, and following the delivery of drugs as well as the vaccine trials as closely as possible. I kept in close contact with my colleagues at HHS, particularly Paul Mango and others involved in tracking and logistics, highly competent people who always knew the current status about medications and vaccines.

Most of my West Wing friends advised me to return to the White House, even to juggle dates between California and Washington, so as to stay under the 130-day limit. Given that the vaccine was developed and my role would be minimal, my distaste for Washington and disgust for the egos and political concerns of the Task Force members won out. The idea of returning was frankly too much to stomach. I decided to resign, rather than head back to Washington for the final few days of my appointment as a special government employee.

After thinking everything through and realizing that my term was running out, I decided to call the president. I dialed the White House operator.

"This is Scott Atlas. Could you please connect me to the president?" I asked. The operator asked me to hold for a moment. Less than a minute later, I heard the familiar voice of one of the receptionists sitting just outside the Oval Office. We exchanged hellos, and she said she would transfer me right in.

"Hello, Scott! How are you?" It was the president. I knew he was on the speakerphone by listening to the sound quality.

"Hi, Mr. President. I am doing well. I hope you are, too." I didn't want to waste time and continued. "I am calling to tell you that I am resigning my position. As you know, my 130-day term as SGE is ending, so I won't be coming back to DC. I wanted to thank you for the opportunity to serve the country and to work with you and your administration."

The president replied, "Thank you, Scott. You did a great job. We had a great relationship. We got a lot done. And you worked hard. You're a fighter. I appreciate that."

"As you know, Mr. President, I always used the latest science to advise you on the best policies to help save lives. We did everything we could to stop the school closures and business closures, even though most states wouldn't reopen," I told him. "And I want to congratulate you on your vision to expedite the vaccine development and drug development under Operation Warp Speed. That was a great accomplishment for the American people. The time line for developing a vaccine was met. We have the vaccine, despite all the obstacles."

The president said, "Thank you, Scott. And I want to tell you something. You were right; you were right about everything."

"Thanks, Mr. President."

He continued. "You were right about everything, all along the way. And you know what? You were also right about something else. Fauci wasn't the biggest problem of all of them. It really wasn't him. You were right about that."

I found myself nodding as I held the phone in my hand. I knew exactly whom he was talking about.

In that moment, the memories flooded back about how the White House, the president, and his closest advisors were ultimately held hostage to the fear of the polling, instead of making the necessary changes to the Task Force. They had let Birx and Fauci tell governors to prolong the lockdowns and school closures and continue the severe restrictions on businesses—strategies that failed to stop the elderly from dying, failed to stop the cases, and destroyed families and sacrificed children. The closest advisors to the president, including the VP, seemed more concerned with politics, even though the Task Force was putting out the wrong advice, contrary to the president's desire to reopen schools and businesses. They had convinced him to do exactly the opposite of what he would naturally do in any other circumstance—to disregard his own common sense and allow grossly incorrect policy advice to prevail. For months, his inner circle feared "rocking the boat" ahead of the election. They stopped the president from getting rid of people who were grossly incompetent, purely because of the election, solely because those highly visible bureaucrats were viewed positively by the public. This president, widely known for his signature "You're fired!" declaration, was misled by his closest political intimates. All for fear of what was inevitable anyway—skewering from an already hostile media. And on top of that tragic misjudgment, the election was lost anyway. So much for political strategists.

So I decided to say it, to be blunt and honest, as I always was with him. I didn't really care about his reaction, even though I was going to insult his most trusted counselors. This had to be said, to set the record straight. And maybe because he was on speakerphone, and I was fully aware his key advisors were probably standing right there, I wanted to say it out loud.

"Well, Mr. President, I will say this. You have balls. I have balls. But the closest people around you—they didn't. They had no balls. They let you down."

I expected but didn't receive any pushback. Instead, he replied quickly, with a slight tone of resignation and acknowledgment in his voice, rather than with any anger.

"Well ... they didn't know, they just didn't know..." and his voice trailed off.

I ended the call with another, "Thank you again." And he repeated, "OK, Scott, we had a great relationship, you did a great job. OK, Scott, good-bye."

I hung up the phone, relieved to have cut all ties to Washington and happy to have spoken the truth, no BS, to the end. Like I told everyone in the White House from early on, I never had any secondary agenda, no motivation other than to do the best I could to help save American lives and to end the tragic, scandalous incompetence. And I would speak the truth, no matter what.

After the call, I immediately emailed and sent in a hard copy of my resignation letter to Staff Secretary Derek Lyons:

THE WHITE HOUSE
WASHINGTON

December 1, 2020

Dear Mr. President:

I am writing to resign from my position as Special Advisor to the President of the United States. I thank you for the honor and privilege to serve on behalf of the American people since August, during these difficult months for our nation. I worked hard with a singular focus – to save lives and help Americans through this pandemic.

As you know, I always relied on the latest science and evidence, without any political consideration or influence. As time went on, like all scientists and health policy scholars, I learned new information and synthesized the latest data from around the world, all in an effort to provide you with the best information to serve the greater public good. But, perhaps more than anything, my advice was always focused on minimizing all the harms from both the pandemic and the structural policies themselves, especially to the working class and the poor.

These views were in agreement with those of many of the world's top epidemiologists and medical scientists from Harvard, Oxford, and other top academic institutions, as well as with those of thousands of medical and public health scientists from around the world. Although some may disagree with those recommendations, it is the free exchange of ideas that lead to scientific truths, which are the very foundation of any civilized society. Indeed, I cannot think of a time where safeguarding science and the scientific debate is more urgent.

Throughout my time at the White House, it was an honor to work with several selfless colleagues in designing specific policies to heighten protection of the vulnerable while safely reopening schools and society. For instance, we increased and prioritized extra personal protective equipment and tens of millions of extra tests to nursing and assisted living facilities, initiated new infection control alliances, implemented more frequent monitoring updates using clinical guidelines to intensify testing, and instituted new outreach to independent seniors in communities. We also successfully designed rational guidelines for safely opening schools, a strategic use of the newly developed testing program, and a national stockpile of drugs for future crises.

We also identified and illuminated early on the harms of prolonged lockdowns, including that they create massive physical health losses and psychological distress, destroy families, and damage our children. And more and more, the relatively low risk to children of serious harms from the infection, the less frequent spread from children, the presence of immunologic protection beyond that shown by antibody testing, and the severe harms from closing schools and society are all being acknowledged.

Mr. President, your Operation Warp Speed team delivered on our promised timelines for new drugs and vaccines. I congratulate you for your vision, and also congratulate the many who did the exemplary work – we know who they are, even though their names are not those familiar to the public.

I sincerely wish the new team all the best as they guide the nation through these trying, polarized times. With the emerging treatments and vaccines, I remain highly optimistic that America will thrive once again and overcome the adversity of the pandemic and all that it has entailed.

Respectfully,

Scott W. Atlas, MD

CHAPTER 19
Assessing the Trump Pandemic Response

I was honored to have served President Trump and the nation in the health crisis of the century. It was a unique privilege to serve on behalf of the American people during those four extremely difficult months for our nation. I worked hard with a singular focus—to save lives and help Americans through the pandemic.

During my time in Washington, as has always been the case, I always relied on the latest science and evidence, without any political consideration or influence. As time went on, like all scientists and health policy scholars, I learned new information and synthesized the latest data from around the world, all in an effort to provide the president and the nation with the best information to serve the greater public good. More than anything, my advice was focused on minimizing the harms from both the pandemic and the policies themselves, especially to the most vulnerable, the working class, and the poor.

My views and policy recommendations were in agreement with those of many of the world's top epidemiologists and medical scientists, as well as tens of thousands of medical and public health scientists from around the world. Although some may disagree with those recommendations, it is the free exchange of ideas that lead to scientific truths, which are the foundation of any civilized society. Indeed, I cannot think of a time where safeguarding science and scientific debate is more urgent. I am forever grateful to the many scientists who counseled me on an almost daily basis to help plow through the emerging research. That was crucial, because scientific journals have become corrupted with poor studies and agenda-based articles. My work also relied on many dedicated people who took the time to carefully analyze the data from around the world, often under duress, to provide real-time answers to my questions. The president and the nation benefitted from their work.

Throughout my time at the White House, it was an honor to work with several selfless colleagues in designing specific policies to heighten protection of the vulnerable while safely reopening schools and society. For instance, we increased and prioritized extra personal protective equipment and tens of millions of extra tests to nursing and assisted-living facilities, initiated new infection control alliances, implemented more frequent monitoring updates using clinical guidelines to intensify testing, and instituted new outreach to independent seniors in communities. These efforts to ramp up protection of the most vulnerable, the elderly in nursing homes, saved lives. In a review published in April 2021, COVID mortality rates in nursing homes declined by almost half, from a high of 20.9 percent in early April to 11.2 percent in early November, without any vaccines. We also successfully designed rational guidelines for safely opening schools, a strategic use of the newly developed testing program, and a national stockpile of drugs for future crises.

I dedicated myself to understanding the pandemic in detail so that I could advise the president and the public on policies that would consider "all health," not just COVID-19. That is the essential demand for any health policy. There is no justification to recommend any policy without considering its potential costs. That is morally and ethically indefensible. Early on, I identified and illuminated the harms of prolonged lockdowns. I am proud to have made the strong case alongside the president for opening in-person schools. More and more, the relatively low risk to children of serious harm from the infection, the less frequent spread from children, the presence of immunologic protection beyond that shown by antibody testing, the efficacy of mitigation measures, and the severe harms from closing schools and society are all being acknowledged.

I arrived in Washington around the end of July 2020. It should be obvious that I was already horrified at our country's response to the crisis—that's why I went to Washington in the first place. For a health policy scholar, there was no more impactful time to apply my work than during the pandemic. And there was nothing more urgently needed than to help my country if asked.

Many assumed that I was there for political reasons. That's false and ignorant. Given their presumptions about me, they thought that I wanted to defend the president and his administration's handling of the pandemic. No one who knows me would believe that. It should be obvious by now that I have zero interest in saying anything that isn't true.

In dozens of interviews while in Washington and since I left, I have been asked to comment on how the United States handled the pandemic. To provide a worthwhile assessment, it's first necessary to clarify the role of the federal government and other levels of government in the management of the SARS2 pandemic. The United States pandemic policy is by design, as follows: a) federally supported, b) state managed, and c) locally implemented. All fifty states independently directed and implemented their own pandemic policies. In every case, governors and local officials were responsible for on-the-ground choices—every business limit, school closing, shelter-in-place order and mask requirement. No policy on any of these issues was set by the federal government, except those involving federal property and employees. What does that mean to the evaluation of a "national strategy" in an enormous country governed by a federalist structure, where states have significant autonomy and responsibilities?

The National "Strategy"

Early on, the president was accused of not having a "strategy" for managing the pandemic. That was a reasonable conclusion, because the overall federal strategy was not at all clear. This lack of clarity was not because the president had failed to articulate a strategy. The appearance of chaos and dysfunction was at least partly due to mixed messages coming out of the White House.

From his March 23, 2020, statement during the initial fifteen-day lockdown that "the cure cannot be worse than the problem," President Trump repeatedly stated his overall strategy: *protect the vulnerable, prevent hospital overcrowding, and open schools and businesses.* These principles were stated numerous times throughout the pandemic in the president's speeches, briefings, and statements issued from inside and outside the White House. Yet focused protection was not implemented by the vast majority of US governors.

The Task Force was called "the White House Coronavirus Task Force," but it was not in synch with President Trump. It was directed by Vice President Pence. He was a thoughtful and engaged participant, and he listened to his main doctors. The medically trained leaders of the White House Task Force were Drs. Fauci and Birx, with an assist from Dr. Robert Redfield, director of the CDC. Drs. Fauci and Birx were very visible to the American public, to the governors, and to all public health officials. They also had a strategy, and they recommended it widely and frequently to the nation. It had one central component: *lockdowns.* That entailed closing schools and businesses; restricting medical care for non-COVID illnesses; testing and quarantining low-risk people; strictly limiting group and family interactions; and restricting personal activities and travel. Almost every governor of every state in the nation implemented it throughout the year and beyond.

I was asked by the president to help at the end of July 2020. For months, I had been stating publicly that the nation was embarking on a hugely incorrect path. The recommendation for prolonged lockdowns was grossly, terribly wrong. That policy was also in direct conflict with the president's own statements advocating reopening schools and businesses. Regardless, the dominant message to the country, pushed by the media and endorsed by what appeared to be most outside experts, was to lock down. School closures, business shutdowns, and a host of restrictions, mandates, and quarantines prevailed throughout the nation. All fifty states closed schools to in-person instruction at some point during the 2019–2020 academic year. Those decisions were all made by the individual governors. Each state had its own variation on the lockdown theme, and local officials then implemented their prescribed lockdown strategy. And, as we know, aside from a few governors, the country did implement and maintain broad lockdowns.

Before assessing the nation's "performance" during the pandemic, this very important and undeniable fact must be clear—with rare exceptions, almost every state in the entire nation implemented and maintained the lockdown policies that were advised by Drs. Fauci and Birx. Any judgment concluding that unnecessary lives were lost due to the failure of the pandemic policies must conclude that the lockdowns failed, because the lockdowns were implemented widely. That is the data.

To be clear, the governors themselves designed, ordered, and controlled their state's lockdowns—the limits on groups, curfews and quarantines, mask mandates, social restrictions, and school and business closures. Those governors followed the advice of Drs. Fauci and Birx, not the advice of others. It is completely wrong and unacceptable that those who advocated for the lockdowns would somehow blame the critics of those lockdowns for the failures of the policy they pushed.

And that policy was a failure, likely the most egregious failure in the history of modern health policy.

The President's Actions—and Inactions

Assigning roles in the pandemic by level of government is a bit more complicated than a straightforward division of responsibilities, because by definition the president himself is the nation's chief executive. Therefore, he has a unique responsibility to lead. He is also the one making the executive decisions. On this highly important criterion of presidential management—taking responsibility to fully take charge of policy coming from the White House—I believe the president made a massive error in judgment. Against his own gut feeling, he delegated authority to medical bureaucrats, and then he failed to correct that mistake.

Why do I conclude that? Because the job of the president is to be the bottom line decision-maker. Of course, he takes advice; he considers the data; he listens to "the experts" and others. And the pandemic is certainly very complicated to understand. No single person has expert-level knowledge about everything that this situation entails. It is absolutely a challenging task to comprehend all aspects of the pandemic in order to formulate appropriate federal policies and recommendations. But there is only one person in charge, and that is supposed to be the president. Decisions on policy for a national emergency are not to be made by a virologist, a public health bureaucrat, a cabinet secretary, or a political advisor. Decisions are not made by committee when there is a chief executive in place. That should go without saying. But that is essentially what happened. The perceived authorities—indeed, the decision-makers—were the president's advisors, Anthony Fauci and Deborah Birx. Even if one accepts that Drs. Fauci and Birx were experts in their fields, they were advisors and nothing more.

Why do I say Fauci and Birx had been given authority beyond their advisory role? Because the president disagreed with the prolonged lockdown strategy. He said it to me repeatedly and made it clear to everyone. He spoke his views to the nation, before and after I arrived. More than a dozen times between spring 2020 and the election, the president specifically spoke about focused protection and reopening. The Birx-Fauci policies were not just directly contrary to the president's statements; the lockdown policies were killing people. But keeping the Task Force intact with its own messaging also did harm to the public. The obvious disconnect between what Fauci and Birx advised and what the president himself advocated sent chaotic mixed messages out of the White House.

Clearly, the largest part of the failure of the president was that he did not change his Task Force. Even before I arrived in Washington as an advisor, there should have been broad personnel changes made in the Task Force. None were made; it remained intact until the end of the president's term. With apologies to true experts, we can quote Churchill, who understood that "nothing would be more fatal than for the Government of States to get in the hands of experts. Expert knowledge is limited knowledge." For an executive widely known for being able to fire people, it was shocking that this president allowed the incompetence of the nation's Task Force advisors to continue.

Dr. Fauci held court in the public eye on a daily basis, so frequently that many misconstrue his role as being in charge. However, it was really Dr. Birx who articulated Task Force policy. All the advice from the Task Force to the states came from Dr. Birx. All written recommendations about their on-the-ground policies were from Dr. Birx. Dr. Birx conducted almost all the visits to states on behalf of the Task Force.

I do not deny that the press made the perception of authority a huge challenge for the president. We all saw how many in the media lionized Drs. Fauci and Birx specifically because of their differences with the president. Communication from the president himself still mattered, however. I strongly believed the president needed to change his personal interaction with the nation. After several awkward press briefings with the Task Force leaders, those briefings had been curtailed. Over the summer, he had become almost invisible. Perhaps because of the conflicts and misstatements at the podium, it seemed the president had decided to remain less visible and delegate to state governors what they all asked for—management of their own state's pandemic. His absence left the public in a state of heightened uncertainty about what the government was doing and what to expect.

That changed substantially after I arrived, because the president decided to resume the briefings. His decision to show the public detailed data on the status of the pandemic changed the mood. Although it wasn't his usual style to do so, he presented statistics on cases, hospitalizations, and deaths in regions, in states, and for the country. The president showed slides and charts on fatality rates and trends, some of which were supplied by the top epidemiologists in the country. He personally communicated on exactly what his government was engaged in—producing and distributing hospital

SCOTT W. ATLAS, MD

equipment, personal protective supplies, tests, ventilators. He described the status of hospital overcrowding, available ICU beds, and
medical personnel. And he provided statistical updates on how the
US was performing, a necessary point of clarification. In fact, the
president was the first to enlighten the press about "excess mortality," by far the most valid statistical basis for such comparisons. The
president's personal role in informing the nation and portraying the
necessary knowledge and attention to detail helped add certainty
and became a success.

The Trump Federal Response

Despite allowing ill-conceived lockdowns to continue being advocated by the Task Force, he president directed several important
and highly successful policies that changed the course of the pandemic and saved lives. To any objective observer, the president and
his administration have a long list of concrete achievements:

- Stopped incoming air travel from China and
  Europe well before other nations, even though
  it was opposed by the Task Force leaders at the
  time.

- Rapidly mobilized and met all requests for extra
  emergency hospital beds and medical personnel for states that thought their hospitals would
  be overwhelmed.

- Invoked the emergency Defense Production
  Act to produce and ship billions of dollars of
  PPE including face shields, gloves, gowns, N95
  and surgical masks, ventilators, and other supplies; the leaders of this effort included names
  the public does not hear, including Federal
  Emergency Management Agency Administrator Pete Gaynor and Admiral John Polowczyk
  of the Supply Chain Stabilization Task Force.

- After a rocky start when it would have been impactful to have far better and more plentiful testing capacity, the administration ultimately devised from scratch and then deployed a massive, state-of-the-art testing apparatus, including advanced antigen tests, point-of-care rapid tests, and an entire array of previously nonexistent technologies.

- Prioritized and then in late summer-fall of 2020, substantially increased the protection of seniors in nursing homes with a multifaceted strategic plan and deliverables, including: intensive testing and hygiene strategies, more than one hundred million N95 masks per month, millions of point-of care rapid tests for all 14,500 certified nursing homes in the nation, new peer-to-peer mentoring in infection-control alliances with nearby hospitals, special CDC strike teams for surge testing when necessary, extra personnel, newly intensive testing requirements for entering staff adjusted to the infection activity in the surrounding communities, and millions of priority pieces of PPE and tests to nonresidential senior centers. All were supported by billions of federal dollars, with performance-based incentives, $250 million for COVID-only facility set-ups, $150 million for infection control assistance, and guidelines for safer visitation to nursing home residents to end isolation from family members. COVID mortality rates in nursing homes declined by almost half, from a high of 20.9 percent in early April to 11.2 percent in early November 2020, before any vaccines.

- Successfully designed rational guidelines for safely opening schools, in concert with physicians, educators, and parents, and supplied massive quantities of extra protective equipment, testing, and other requirements to states in order to remove all obstacles to opening in-person schools.

- Operation Warp Speed removed nearly all financial risk from the private sector by betting on American ingenuity and hit on all promised time lines. The administration allocated billions of dollars for purchasing hundreds of millions of doses before vaccine approval, as well as prioritizing production materials, facilitating delivery, and taking full responsibility for vaccine administration to patients. OWS accelerated and developed highly effective vaccines for emergency use authorization in record time, shocking all experts by delivering them within hours after EUA using advanced preparation of logistics in less than one year, a process that normally takes about four or five years, and then starting injection into the highest risk elderly in December 2020.

- Operation Warp Speed accelerated more than forty clinical trials for the development of several novel drug treatments for emergency use authorization (EUA) in partnership with several pharmaceutical companies that improved outcomes, reduced lengths of hospital stays, and markedly reduced risk of hospitalization. These drugs were produced in record time, including monoclonal antibody treatments and other advanced technology agents.

- By mid-December 2020, the federal government had expedited logistics and delivered these lifesaving drugs, including novel antibody treatments that reduce hospitalizations of high-risk elderly by more than 70 percent. According to HHS, more than two hundred thousand doses of these monoclonal-antibody drugs had been delivered to hospitals in all fifty states by December 2020.

- Created a national strategic stockpile of important drugs, protective equipment, and logistics to help in future pandemics.

- Turned around the nation during the pandemic with the fastest-rebounding economy in the world before leaving office.

Operation Warp Speed

As I write this book, high-risk Americans and people all over the world are benefitting from the vaccines and therapies developed under President Trump's Operation Warp Speed. In record time, several vaccines were developed, produced, distributed, and administered. Many who did this exemplary work for the American people have not received the credit due. Those of us inside the White House know who they are, even though their names are not familiar to the public. A very incomplete list includes:

- Alex Azar, Secretary of Health and Human Services and CEO of the OWS program, who was the architect of the business plan and of creating a separate governance process.

- Moncef Slaoui, Chief Scientific Officer and the one who created the portfolio of vaccines in which we invested.

- General Gus Perna, Chief Operating Officer, the logistician who designed the entire vaccine delivery program. Also, very instrumental in securing raw materials and equipment from all over the world to set up production facilities and factories.

- Lt. General Paul Ostrowski, Director of Supply, Production, and Distribution for OWS, who worked alongside General Perna to execute the plan for the manufacture, distribution, and administration of approved therapeutics and vaccines valued at over $16 billion, including hundreds of millions of doses and more than forty thousand vaccination centers throughout the country.

- Carlo de Notaristefani, Lead Advisor for Manufacturing and Supply Chain at Operation Warp Speed, the manufacturing expert who helped stand up and equip twenty-five manufacturing locations.

- Francis Collins, Director of the NIH, who designed the clinical trials and brought together a leadership team from the entire industry to help him.

- Matt Hepburn, director of Department of Defense's OWS activities, who served both General Perna and Dr. Slaoui managing the vaccine-development program.

- Janet Woodcock, Therapeutics Lead for OWS, who led the development and introduction of monoclonal antibodies and other treatments.

- Dr. Robert Kadlec, Assistant Secretary for Preparedness and Response, HHS, who months before formal launch of OWS began ordering a billion needles, syringes, and vials for vaccine delivery.

- Paul Mango, senior advisor to Secretary Azar, kept me informed every step of the way, so that I would never misspeak or transmit any inaccurate information to the president of the United States about vaccines or drugs under OWS.

History will undoubtedly malign many of the Trump administration's activities and its legacy, but it will be very difficult to deny the accomplishments of Operation Warp Speed. While I personally cannot take credit for it, I am proud to have been part of the administration that devised such an important and successful government program, one that saved countless lives. Regardless of the ongoing controversies about the use of the vaccines in populations without serious risk from COVID and the inappropriate vaccine mandates, their development and distribution were a remarkable triumph of public policy, a true partnership between government and the private sector.

CHAPTER 20
And That's the Science!

"They're never going to admit they were wrong."

Governor Ron DeSantis

DeSantis: Florida vs. Lockdowns; May 29, 2021

In any health crisis, the underpinning of policymaking is the evidence at hand. It was also essential to apply simple common sense and logic. Unfortunately, logic is not part of the curriculum in science departments. Apparently, neither is critical thinking.

We knew who was at risk to die. We knew who was not. Millions of people were carrying the virus by the spring. Why wouldn't we protect those at risk, instead of locking down the healthy and destroying everyone, a strategy that, by the way, was failing to protect those at risk?

Instead of emphasizing the large body of empirical data already gathered, our public health leaders and media kept predictions of mathematical models front and center, highlighted to the public in headline after headline. Predictive models for analyzing complex problems are extremely valuable, no doubt. Oxford University Professor Sunetra Gupta, one of the world's most renowned epidemiologists and modelers, authored a 2001 piece in *Nature* subtitled "Scientists sometimes use mathematics to give the illusion of certainty." In the article she wrote, "Mathematics—which has proved to be an indispensable tool in scientific inquiry—distinguishes itself by the lack of ambiguity in its terms. Mathematical metaphors are powerful analytical tools precisely because of the unequivocal relationships between their components." She went on, "Of greater concern is that, when one is attempting to formalize a set of complicated interactions, assumptions can creep in unawares.... It is unfortunate that the assumptions embedded in the mathematical structures employed may not always be obvious to the general public."

Sunetra's prescient warning that "no phoenix is likely to arise out of the ashes of a misguided mathematical model" went unheeded. Models with severely flawed assumptions were relied upon far too long despite their failures. Even on simple analysis, COVID-19 models had already demonstrated wild variations in their projections. As just one example, predictions for number of US deaths only three weeks later with eight different models, as analyzed by COVID-19 Forecast Hub on June 3, 2020, ranged from 2,419 to 11,190—a 4.5-fold difference.

It was not only the remarkable variability of the models that should have limited their use as tools for policy. Detailed analyses had already shown massive failures in their predictions. One of the most egregious cases—and perhaps the one most to blame for causing government officials to introduce the lockdowns—were the wildly alarmist predictions from the Imperial College model of Neil Ferguson and colleagues. For Sweden, the Imperial College model predicted 30,434 deaths if under lockdowns, and 66,393 deaths if left unmitigated; after a full year of ignoring Ferguson's strategy, as of March 2021, Sweden had a total of 13,496 deaths. In addition to its outlandish projections for the UK, the US, and most other countries, one review in July 2020 showed the model had also severely overprojected mortality associated with reopening in all five US states it had included.

As Stanford University's Ioannidis, University of Sydney's Cripps, and Northwestern's Tanner documented in August 2020, forecasts built directly on significant data at hand also fared poorly. As one example, a Massachusetts General Hospital model predicted over 23,000 deaths within a month of Georgia's reopening—the actual deaths were 896. The University of Washington's Institute for Health Metrics and Evaluation (IHME) was wildly off in its May 3, 2020, predictions of Sweden's deaths to rise to 494 only three weeks later—an overestimate by a multiple of eight times!

Models had also failed in predictions about ICU bed utilizations, as the frequently cited IHME model had done. Projections made only twenty-four hours in advance of the day in question were also far off. Four models were analyzed for their accuracy to predict COVID deaths by state for the following day. For most states, the models' projections were outside their own standard errors of estimates more than 80 percent of the time, *even for next-day death predictions.*

In their August 2020 review of several models, Ioannidis, Cripps, and Tanner lamented what other leaders in the field had similarly expressed, "In fact, it is surprising that epidemic forecasting has retained much credibility among decision-makers, given its dubious track record."

Regardless of the obvious and continual failures of statistical models, the prominent display of those same models in the media continued. Why? One factor was undoubtedly that vastly inaccurate predictions suffered no serious consequences. I also think that too many anointed experts had already publicly declared their allegiance to those models. The discussion about models represents one of the early displays of *groupthink* in this pandemic. The repetition of misinformation from many voices became accepted as truth. Media outlets and prominent policymakers clung to those same failed models, and they kept inciting panic. No truer words were written than the warning by Ioannidis, Cripps, and Tanner back in August 2020—"It is not just an issue of academic debate, it is an issue of potentially devastating, wrong decisions."

Bottom line: projections from mathematical models about the SARS2 pandemic predicting doomsday scenarios used faulty assumptions and were generally highly inaccurate. That's the science.

Children and COVID-19

One important concern about a fatal infection would obviously be the risk of death to children. A striking feature of this virus was that it spared almost all children from death and serious illness. This fact is unquestionably critical to the design of the best policies to protect individuals and families. Yet it remained nearly unstated by the American media for many months; that scientific fact was even actively refuted.

I spoke publicly about the extraordinarily low risk to children early and often, beginning in the spring of 2020 and throughout the year. After analyzing the world's data and the early New York City data, where a third of deaths in the US pandemic had occurred, I listed their April 2020 statistics that showed the rate of death for people under eighteen years old was zero per 100,000. In New York City in the 2020 summer, 99.94 percent of deaths occurred in people over eighteen; only one child without underlying conditions died, comprising 0.005 percent of 18,988 deaths. As of February 10, 2021, only 137 of 443,107 (0.03 percent) of total CDC-documented COVID-19 deaths were in children under fifteen; only 763 (0.17 percent) were in those under twenty-five. CDC later calculated those under twenty to have a 99.997 percent chance of survival. John Ioannidis, renowned Stanford epidemiologist, summed it up well almost a year ago—the risk of dying for young people from COVID-19 is "almost zero."

It was also clearly shown that young adults and children in normal health have an extremely low risk of *any* serious illness from COVID-19. Hospitalizations in young children from COVID, a reflection of serious illness, are far less frequent than in adults, by a factor of twenty times to over one hundred times less, depending on age. CDC reported that hospitalization rates for those eighteen to twenty-nine are very small compared to older age groups. Exceptions existed, as they do with virtually every other clinically encountered infection, but that should not outweigh the overwhelming evidence to the contrary.

A media frenzy erupted in late spring 2020 about a rare complication associated with COVID-19 in children, multisystem inflammatory syndrome, similar to Kawasaki disease. The sensationalistic reporting confused the public, because the association is very uncommon. Again, no medical perspective was offered by the key public health officials to a fearful public on the news. Just like the rare Kawasaki disease, affecting only 3,000 to 5,000 children in the United States each year, at the time of this writing a similar number has been reported with COVID. The syndrome is an exception, typically treatable, and it never has been regarded previously as a risk so serious that schools must be shuttered.

The medical science was consistent from the early days of the pandemic that even seasonal influenza is more dangerous to young children than this coronavirus. This perspective would have been enormously reassuring to parents, yet it was never put forth by those dominating the public narrative. For months, I quoted the *JAMA Pediatrics* study of forty-six North American pediatric hospitals that flatly stated in the summer of 2020, "Our data indicate that children are at far greater risk of critical illness from influenza than from COVID-19." Children are also more frequently hospitalized from the flu and transmit the flu widely to high-risk adults, who die every season from the flu to the tune of 35,000 to 90,000 in the US alone. It was met with media silence when the CDC concurred in the fall of 2020 that "in this pandemic, deaths of children are less than in each of the last five flu seasons," when about 200 or more children die every winter. One case in point is California, where 5.4 percent of its 2017–2018 flu deaths were in children. For California COVID deaths, as of June 9, 2021, *0 percent* of 62,538 Californians who died were children under eighteen, even though they make up 13 percent of California's total COVID cases. Of the 481,576 cases of infection in children under eighteen in California, 23 died as of June 9, 2021; that means 99.996 percent of kids who caught the infection survived.

Bottom line: from the world's data, we know that children have had an extremely low risk for any serious illness from COVID-19 and no significant risk of death. That's the science.

Even if children have not themselves been at any significant risk from this illness, what about those at high-risk in multigenerational homes or who are in contact with children in schools? Did children transmit COVID-19? Most parents and teachers understand that young children are often significant spreaders of the flu and the common cold.

This was not influenza, though. Although not necessary to justify reopening schools, it was well documented from studies all over the world that almost all SARS2 coronavirus transmission to children comes from adults, and not the other way around. The earliest study was a carefully done, highly sophisticated, molecular contact tracing study that systematically traced every case from Iceland in the April 2020 *New England Journal of Medicine*. That study's senior author concluded that "even if children do get infected, they are less likely to transmit the disease to others than adults. *We have not found a single instance of a child infecting parents.*" (emphasis added). That fact, that kids don't transmit COVID to adults frequently if at all, seemed to be the icing on the cake to the case for reopening in-person schools.

That children only rarely transmit the infection to adults was verified in multiple contact tracing and other scientific studies, including independent data from more than a dozen countries in Europe, including a Swiss study showing that school was the source of only 0.3 percent of the infections. Moreover, teachers are not at higher risk of COVID-19 compared with other professions and do not have a significant risk of becoming infected from children in school, proven over a year ago. In one study that inspired harassment and threats to its author when it was eventually published in the *NEJM*, Sweden kept its schools open throughout their pandemic surge, without mask-wearing or social-distancing mandates. They experienced an extremely low incidence of significant COVID-19 and zero deaths in nearly 2 million school children ages one to sixteen. Sweden's teachers showed no increase in age-adjusted risk of severe COVID-19. The European Centre for Disease Prevention reported a seventeen-country study and concluded that "[open] schools were not associated with accelerating community transmission."

One would think these scientific discoveries would be welcomed with tremendous joy. They were not. The media played its role in purveying fear, as did our public health leaders. A surge of cases in Israel last summer was first reported to correlate with school reopening. Tabloid-like headlines and articles generated intense fear in parents and policymakers, blaring across the world in July 2020 that Israel's school reopening was "a disaster," "a cautionary tale," and catastrophic.

One problem—that conclusion was false. My own detailed analysis of Israel's mobility data, helped by fantastic digging by some talented and tenacious analysts on whom I often relied, showed that Israel had returned to pre-pandemic social mingling before school reopening. That fact has since been independently verified, recently published in the scientific literature in January 2021—yet the false conclusion that blamed the surge on schools was never corrected in the media. A South Korea contact tracing study also generated false, alarming headlines in the *New York Times*. The corrected analysis showing no evidence of a child passing the infection to an adult was never reported.

Bottom line: Months before the fall 2020 school year, the overwhelming weight of scientific data showed the risk of transmission of SARS2 from children to adults is extremely small. There is no special risk to teachers in schools; in fact, schools are a low-risk environment. That's the science.

* * * * *

What about school closures? Three undeniable realities formed the basis of my policy advice to reopen in-person schools. First, children do not have significant risk of serious illness or death from this virus. Second, the harms to children of closing in-person schooling are dramatic and irrefutable, including poor learning, dropouts, social isolation, suicidal ideation, most of which are far worse for lower-income groups. Third, as I wrote in July 2020, "Educating is not just an 'essential business'; it is at the top of the list of our nation's priorities." A fourth important fact, one not necessary to justify reopening schools, was well-documented from studies all over the world that almost all coronavirus transmission to children comes from adults, not the other way around. Science overwhelmingly supported opening in-person K-12 schools more than a year ago. It is false to claim that new information since the fall of 2020 suddenly indicated that schools should reopen.

I had little doubt that those with affluence and privilege had the means to compensate for closed schools, but that did not apply to the rest of the country. The Northwest Evaluation Association (NWEA), an education research association, called attention to drops in reading and math learning of up to 50 percent from spring school closures, with low-income kids having the largest drops. A study in fall 2020 from Stanford's Center for Research on Education Outcomes demonstrated substantial learning losses from the spring 2020 school closures alone. They introduced their results with the statement: "First, the findings [on learning losses] are chilling."

An explosion of failing grades began accumulating, underscoring the total failure of online education. First-quarter grades in the fall of 2020 in Fairfax County, Virginia, public schools showed F-marks increased by 83 percent. The increase in students receiving two F-grades was 300 percent for middle school students, especially in female students (600 percent increase), Hispanic students (400 percent increase), students with disabilities (400 percent increase), English-learner students (383 percent increase) and economically disadvantaged students (375 percent increase). The increase in high school students receiving two F-grades was 50 percent.

School closures were especially harmful to children in lower-income and less-educated households, who often depend on school services that affluent families do not. The CDC July 2020 report had acknowledged that "disparities in education outcomes caused by school closures are a particular concern for low-income and minority students and students with disabilities." Researchers associated with the Centre for Economic Policy Research summarized last fall that "school and childcare closures have significant negative long-term consequences on the human capital and welfare of the affected children, especially those from disadvantaged socioeconomic backgrounds." It was commonly acknowledged that school closures would further the gaps between lower-income and minority kids and kids from higher-income families, quantifiable disparities that would likely last.

Extraordinarily harmful, nonacademic damages are also inflicted on children by extended school closures, and they were well known by the summer of 2020. The CDC listed some, including harms to the development of social and emotional skills: "Being in a school setting with peers and teachers is also associated with lower levels of depression, thoughts about suicide, social anxiety, and sexual activity, as well as higher levels of self-esteem and more adaptive use of free time."

In just two months of school closures in March and April of 2020, a Florida study estimated that approximately 15,000 child abuse cases went unreported, or 27 percent fewer than expected for these two months. The authors admitted that their number was "likely underestimated" but noted that for the United States, their conservative calculation would imply 212,500 unreported child abuse cases in those two months of school closures alone. In New York City, thousands of cases of child maltreatment went unreported during the spring 2020 school closures, according to research published in the scientific journal *Child Abuse and Neglect*. Researchers reported a 29 percent to more than 50 percent drop in referrals to children's agencies during March, April, and May—because schools represent the number one agency where neglect and child abuse are noted.

The CDC also published in July 2020 that one in four of America's college-aged kids contemplated suicide after the first three months of lockdowns. Almost three-fourths of those aged eighteen to twenty-four reported at least one mental-health symptom by the end of June, with doubling or tripling in symptoms of anxiety and depressive disorders. The National Bureau of Economic Research reported that the most fearful age group of all was the eighteen- to thirty-four-year-olds, those with by far the smallest risk from the illness, grossly overestimating their extraordinarily small risk of death or serious illness by several orders of magnitude. And more recently, the American Psychological Association reported that 52 percent of eighteen- to twenty-four-year-olds experienced an unwanted weight gain over the lockdown, averaging a shocking twenty-eight pounds; another 22 percent had a large unwanted weight loss over twenty pounds. YouGov reported that a full 50 percent of college-aged Americans said in March 2021 they now "feel nervous" about any social interactions with other people, almost double that of elderly Americans who have far more risk from the illness. The strict lockdowns generated a tripling of visits to doctors by American teenagers for self-harm, things like wrist slashing, personal body mutilation, or other forms of self-in-flicted abuse.

In spite of the overwhelming body of scientific evidence and in disregard of the massive physical, psychological, and emotional harms to America's children, only 17 percent of 14,944 school districts studied were fully open for in-person instruction in the fall term of 2020, according to the CDC in *JAMA Pediatrics*. According to Burbio's data on 1,200 districts, including the 200 largest school districts in the US, over 60 percent of US students were attending schools that were virtual-only in September 2020. At the college level, too, those running America's universities from coast to coast also failed our younger generation and kept closing campuses.

Yet lo and behold, after the election, the compelling case to open all schools in-person was admitted by many journalists, even in publications that had been touting the lockdown line for months: "Trump has been demanding for months that schools reopen, and on that he seems to have been largely right," Nicholas Kristof wrote on November 18, 2020, in the *New York Times* while exposing his own politicized framing of the issue. "Schools, especially elementary schools, do not appear to have been major sources of coronavirus transmission, and remote learning is proving to be a catastrophe for many low-income children."

On January 28, 2021, the *Atlantic*, went further in "The Truth about Kids, School, and COVID-19," openly admitting that the case to reopen schools was longstanding truth: "Research from around the world has, *since the beginning of the pandemic* [emphasis added], indicated that people under 18, and especially younger kids, are less susceptible to infection, less likely to experience severe symptoms, and far less likely to be hospitalized or die.... We've known for months that young children are less susceptible to serious infection and less likely to transmit the coronavirus. Let's act like it."

In continuation of their malfeasance, some government officials falsely claimed they are "open" while being in-person for only one or two days per week. Not until the end of April 2021 did even 50 percent of US school districts offer fully in-person learning, according to American Enterprise Institute and Davidson College reporting. My current state, California, stands strong when it comes to K-12 schools—as the most science-denying state in the nation. The lowest index of in-person schooling in the nation was held by California's public schools. By Burbio's calculation, less than 17 percent of California's students were in fully in-person schools as of June 2021. That compares to Florida, where 100 percent of students had fully in-person schools for the entire academic year since fall 2020. Nationally, 55 percent of students are enrolled in schools with fully in-person classes; 45 percent are not.

Bottom line: The policy of reopening in-person schools has been supported by the data, time after time, for more than a full year. And the United States stands out, in abject shame even among our peer nations since the fall of 2020, uniquely willing to sacrifice its children out of fear for adults. And that's the science.

The Painful Truth about Masks

In many ways, there is nothing more representative of the SARS2 coronavirus pandemic than masks. After initially being dismissed on the basis of published science and empirical evidence, masks abruptly became a topic discussed with a fervor normally reserved for religion. Even today, after the overwhelming empirical evidence from all over the world, conclusive research studies with solid experimental design published in scientific journals, and revelations from newly visible emails unveiling truths previously denied, masks remain one of the most polarizing topics of all. More than anything else, the residual radioactivity around the mask discussion illustrates the strength of human resistance to relinquishing a dearly held belief, even in the face of clear-cut evidence to the contrary. That is why masks are still the "third rail" of this pandemic.

Belief in the efficacy of masks was supported by at least one simple observation. Doctors, I often heard in rebuttal, wear masks! Indeed, in all the hundreds of medical procedures I had performed,

I wore a surgical mask. But the real reason doctors wear masks is to stop large droplets of saliva, coughs, or sneezes from entering the sterile field and contaminating a wound or incision. They do not wear masks in operating rooms to stop aerosolized viruses emitted via breathing.

This virus primarily spreads by aerosols, invisible with every breath. That type of spread escapes around a mask. That's why you see your sunglasses fog up even though you wear a mask, just like breath travels around a face shield or a plastic barrier between restaurant tables. "COVID-19 is being increasingly recognised as an airborne disease, meaning that the virus can fluctuate in the air, like a gas," according to the *British Medical Journal* in an attempt to explain why masks should not even be expected to block this virus.

We also know that it passes through the holes of the surgical mask. Dr. Fauci, in his publicly uncovered email to Sylvia Burwell, former secretary of HHS, explained the reality to his former colleague: "The typical mask you buy in the drug store is not really effective in keeping out a virus, which is small enough to pass through the material. It might, however, provide some slight benefit in keeping out gross droplets if someone coughs or sneezes on you." The SARS2 virus is about 0.12 microns in size, similar to influenza and far smaller than the pore size in surgical masks. It should not be necessary to explain how absurd it was to even consider that a scarf or bandana would stop the virus.

Nevertheless, I was warned by several prominent medical scientists, well-meaning colleagues, and friends that I should stay silent about masks. Their rationale was based on the idea that people would never accept evidence that masks are not effective. They told me people desperately needed to feel like they had some control, and the simple face covering, absurd pseudoscience or not, provided it. If that illusion was taken away, then a feeling of total helplessness would be the natural conclusion. They were absolutely certain that I would provoke a mountain of hate and worse, even though I would be stating the truth. The backlash was inevitable, and powerful people would be embarrassed, they warned.

I personally wished that masks worked. But for several important reasons, I pushed back on mask mandates requiring general mask usage in society. I could not endorse a requirement for unscientific, irrational behavior. I do not choose to wear a copper bracelet for arthritis. Others may choose to, and that's fine. I am in favor of having everyone who wants a mask to wear one.

I had written and advised many times that symptomatic people should isolate and wear masks when others were nearby. I also consistently and explicitly recommended in dozens of publications and national media interviews to "wear a mask when you cannot socially distance." That provides some protection against infectious droplets, as in coughs or sneezes. My words echoed those of the Harvard Medical School authors of the *NEJM* article "Universal Masking in Hospitals in the Covid-19 Era," which are featured at the very top of that page: "On June 3, 2020, the authors of this article state "We strongly support the calls of public health agencies for all people to wear masks when circumstances compel them to be within 6 ft of others for sustained periods." I had even written in April 2020, "Masks could be required for public transit" owing to those tight spaces, while also acknowledging that people would want to feel safe or they wouldn't reenter society.

I recommended that masks be used for symptomatic patients and for those caring for them, particularly when near high-risk individuals. For coughing or sneezing, as symptomatic patients might do, I knew that a mask would at least block large droplets with infectious material, and a confined space would be a setup for that. That matches the very precise wording of the National Institutes of Health. In their December 17, 2020, update, they specified, "When consistent distancing is not possible, face coverings may further reduce the spread of infectious droplets from individuals with SARS-CoV-2 infection to others." "When consistent distancing is not possible…"—and note the absence of mentioning reducing the spread other than by droplets.

That recommendation was very different, though, from having everyone walking around outside wearing a mask. Masks were already proven to be ineffective for influenza, a virus of similar size. That had been reviewed by the CDC in May 2020 and by Oxford University's Centre for Evidence-Based Medicine in July 2020. The empirical evidence from the US and all over the world already had shown masks failed to stop COVID-19 cases from surging. Chart after chart refuted the claim that masks stopped the spread of cases. It seemed strange for outdoor mask mandates to be considered, when data had shown that cases spread with far greater chances indoors, in households, not outside in open spaces. Yet even today, in the summer of 2021, the Stanford University community is filled with young, healthy people wearing masks outside, on their bikes, in their cars, jogging in the fresh air.

Masks were harmful, too. It was not simply the long-published lists of biological and practical harms written by the WHO and others, still denied by the most strenuous of mask zealots. Relying on masks would be dangerous, implying protection for those at risk to die, like the vulnerable elderly, when legitimate protection was not conferred. Requiring masks would also increase the fear, as a visible public reminder of the "extreme danger." In June 2021, the dangers of masks in children were finally suggested publicly in *JAMA Pediatrics*; harmful accumulations of carbon dioxide were noted even in short-term mask wearing. Masks impede communication and create a poor learning environment in school; bacterial contamination occurs, especially with longer use; masks cause eye and skin infections. All and more are documented in dozens of scientific publications and reports, as outlined by the UK's Professor Ellen Townsend and others. The WHO acknowledged it by recommending against masks during exercise. And does any person honestly believe that children's psychological development will be unaffected after being imprinted with the idea that everyone, including themselves, poses a constant danger to everyone else?

Let's look at what was scientifically known back in the spring-summer of 2020:

- In April 2020, *New England Journal of Medicine* published a study on universal masking for health care workers. The Harvard Medical School authors began by stating what was known: "We know that wearing a mask outside health care facilities offers little, if any, protection from infection.... In many cases, the desire for widespread masking is a reflexive reaction to anxiety over the pandemic."

- The CDC in May 2020 published a thorough review of influenza pandemics and concluded "(we) did not find evidence that surgical-type face masks are effective in reducing laboratory-confirmed influenza transmission, either when worn by infected persons (source control) or by persons in the general community to reduce their susceptibility."

- In WHO's June 2020 "Advice on the Use of Masks in the Context of COVID-19," they summarized by stating, "At present, there is no direct evidence (from studies on COVID19 and in healthy people in the community) on the effectiveness of universal masking of healthy people in the community to prevent infection with respiratory viruses, including COVID-19" and "there are potential benefits and harms to consider" in December 2020, as well.

- On July 23, 2020, Tom Jefferson and Carl Heneghan of University of Oxford's Centre for Evidence-Based Medicine reviewed the scientific literature and wrote, "It would appear that despite two decades of pandemic preparedness, there is considerable uncertainty as to the value of wearing masks."

- In November 2020, Jefferson published another thorough review of the data on masks in influenza, a virus of similar size to SARS2, entitled "Physical interventions to interrupt or reduce the spread of respiratory viruses." From nine published trials he concluded "results of randomised trials did not show a clear reduction in respiratory viral infection with the use of medical/surgical masks during seasonal influenza."

Beyond those summaries of research in respiratory viruses, a large amount of empirical evidence accumulated from all over the world about masks for COVID-19. That evidence—based in real-life experience—was clear and consistent. Mask usage failed to stop or prevent surges in cases in dozens of cities, states, and countries.

- In the US, thirty-eight states had mandates for masks since the summer of 2020, and most of the others had mask mandates in their major cities. By early fall the failure of mask wearing to prevent surging COVID cases was shown from coast to coast and beyond—Hawaii, California, Georgia, LA County, Miami-Dade County, Alabama, and more. And don't be fooled by false claims about American disobedience. Data from Gallup, YouGov, the Covid-19 Consortium, the CDC, and elsewhere showed that approximately 80 percent or more of Americans had been wearing masks since the late summer of 2020, equal to or surpassing most Western European nations and approaching the levels in Asia. There was no evidence that masks stopped surges in cases.

Dr. Redfield testified to Congress that "if every one of us (wore a mask), this pandemic would be over in eight to 12 weeks"—and this set of charts shows how false that is:

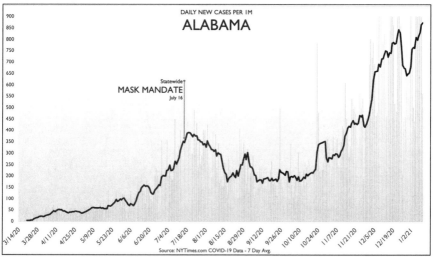

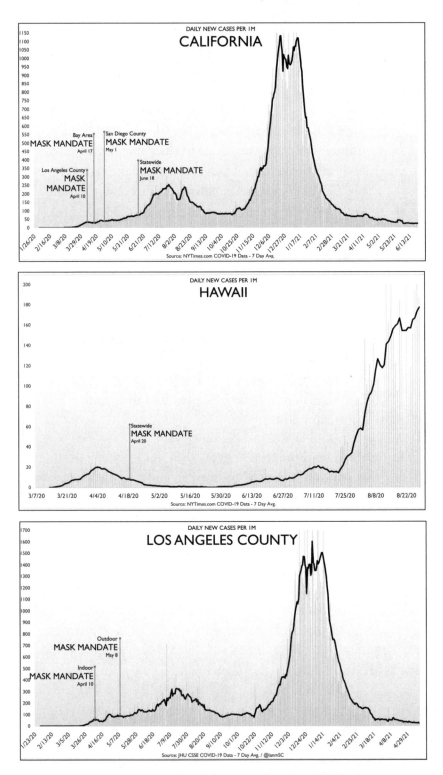

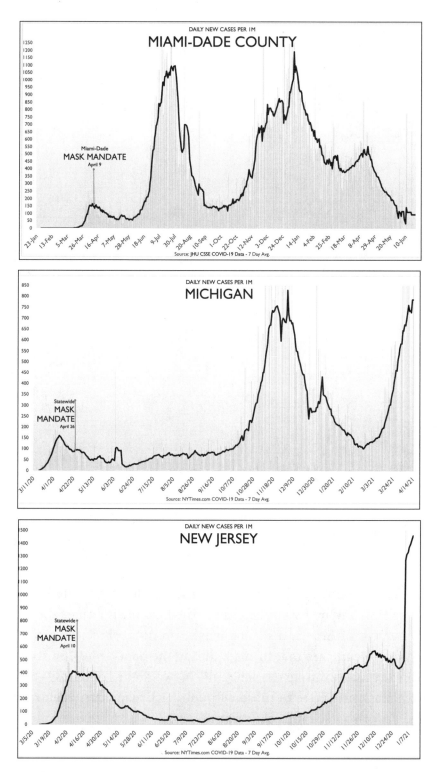

289

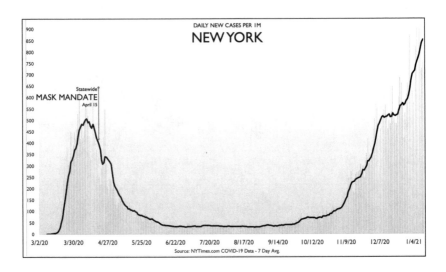

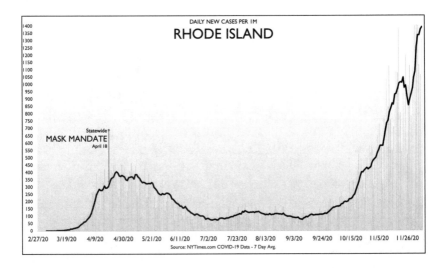

What about the effectiveness of masks for the United States overall? Below are two more charts. The first one is a chart showing 80 percent of Americans using masks (in dots) since the summer of 2020—compare that to cases during the pandemic. The second compares cases during the pandemic in two groups of states—those with mask mandates to those without mask mandates. Feel free to decide for yourself if masks stopped cases!

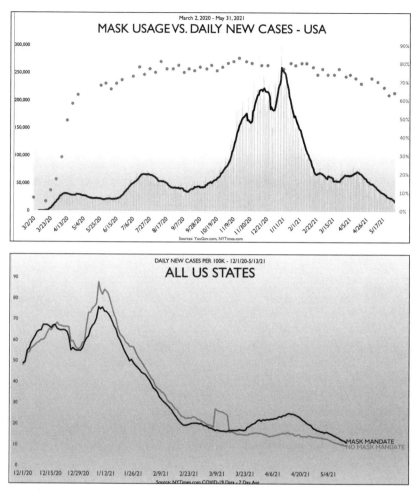

Outside the US, countries far and wide had long implemented mask mandates, and they too were wearing them. Yet cases surged through those mandates. I wondered how these surges, so simple to observe and document, somehow remained so invisible. It certainly was not hard to find examples from spring-summer-fall of 2020—Austria, Belgium, France, Germany, Israel, Italy, Japan, Portugal, Spain, and the UK, just for a start. In South Korea, when a full 99 percent of people were wearing masks for months, cases exploded though their police-enforced mask mandates.

Perhaps masks stopped COVID cases in other countries, maybe because Americans just would not wear masks? This set of charts shows how false that is:

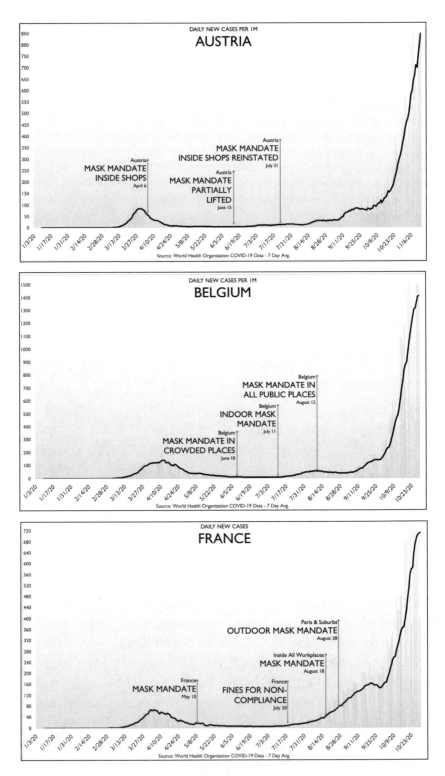

DAILY NEW CASES PER 1M
AUSTRIA

Austria†
MASK MANDATE
INSIDE SHOPS REINSTATED
July 21

Austria†
MASK MANDATE
INSIDE SHOPS
April 6

Austria†
MASK MANDATE
PARTIALLY
LIFTED
June 15

Source: World Health Organization COVID-19 Data - 7 Day Avg.

DAILY NEW CASES PER 1M
BELGIUM

Belgium†
MASK MANDATE IN
ALL PUBLIC PLACES
August 12

Belgium†
INDOOR MASK
MANDATE
July 11

Belgium†
MASK MANDATE IN
CROWDED PLACES
June 10

Source: World Health Organization COVID-19 Data - 7 Day Avg.

DAILY NEW CASES
FRANCE

Paris & Suburbs†
OUTDOOR MASK MANDATE
August 28

Inside All Workplaces†
MASK MANDATE
August 18

France†
MASK MANDATE
May 10

France†
FINES FOR NON-
COMPLIANCE
July 20

Source: World Health Organization COVID-19 Data - 7 Day Avg.

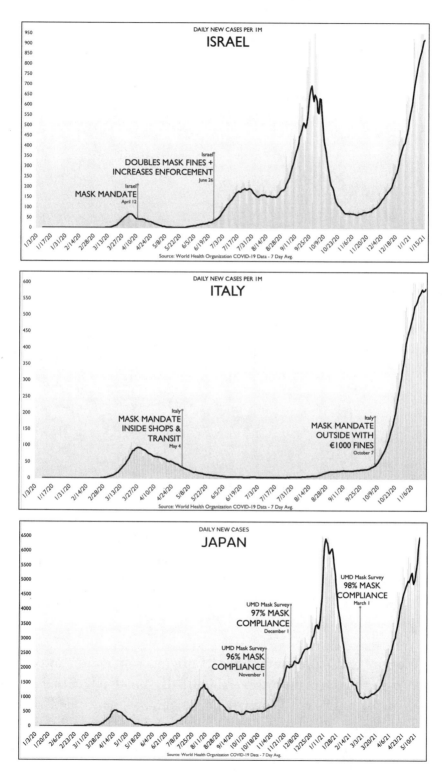

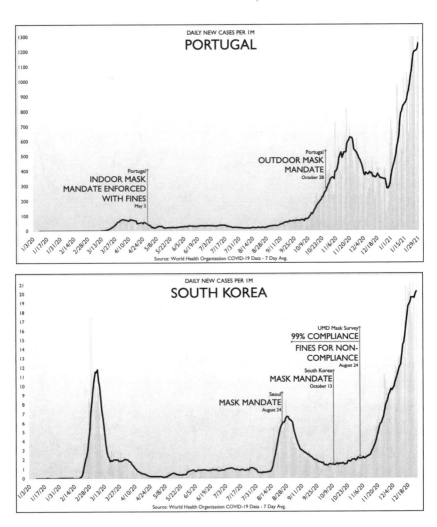

In sum, the evidence shows that masks did not control rises in infections from COVID-19. Yet anyone questioning the efficacy of broad mask mandates was subjected to vilification and outright censorship.

* * * * *

In November 2020, months after its original submission and difficult-to-justify rejection by several journals, *Annals of Internal Medicine* finally published Denmark's "randomized, controlled" Danmask-19 study. That seminal study—of the highest scientific quality in clinical trial research—evaluated masks in more than 6,000 adult participants. That study showed there was no statistically significant difference between those who wore masks and those who did not when it came to being infected by the SARS2 coronavirus—nothing different between masks and no masks.

For those who want the details: Of those wearing masks, 1.8 percent caught the infection, compared to 2.1 percent of the control group not wearing masks, with a p-value of 0.33 (that means there is no significant difference between the groups). If you only look at people who said they wore masks "exactly as instructed," this did not make any difference to the results; there was no difference between mask wearers and those without masks (p=0.40). The results of the Danmask-19 trial confirmed all reviews about the lack of effectiveness of population masks in influenza. Likewise, for all eleven respiratory viruses other than SARS2, there was no significant difference between mask wearers and those who did not wear a mask. The Denmark study used high-quality surgical masks. The bottom line of the Denmark study is clear—*masks did not reduce the incidence of infection from SARS2 or any other virus.*

Oxford's Heneghan and Jefferson explained the unique importance of the Danish research. The only previous reports that had claimed masks to be effective at stopping airborne diseases had been "observational"—not solid, scientifically valid research. Studies like that observed people who used masks, relied on anecdotal reporting and memory, and had no randomized control group for a valid comparison. Other reports, like the hairdresser publication posted by the CDC, were not remotely close to generating scientifically valid conclusions, owing to several serious flaws in design. Particle model studies were held up by others, because many showed masks stop certain particles—that does not mean they stop the spread of a contagious viral infection. All good scientists understood these flaws. Heneghan and Jefferson emphasized to finally, unequivocally settle the mask issue: "Now that we have properly rigorous scientific research we can rely on, the evidence shows that wearing masks in the community does not significantly reduce the rates of infection."

To add nails to the coffin, in May 2021 University of Louisville researchers published a detailed analysis of the effectiveness of masks and mask mandates in United States, using CDC data covering multiple seasons during the 2020 pandemic. The bottom line conclusion was "Our main finding is that mask mandates and use are not associated with lower SARS-CoV-2 spread among US states." They found that "80% of US states mandated masks during the COVID-19 pandemic. Those mandates induced greater mask compliance, but did not predict lower growth rates when community spread was low or high."

There is no ambiguity in the Louisville researchers' conclusion. "In summary, mask mandates and [mask] use were poor predictors of COVID-19 spread in US states…. Our findings do not support the hypothesis that SARS-CoV-2 transmission rates decrease with greater public mask use."

Perhaps the clearest indication of the deeply damaged psyche of many Americans is their refusal to accept that masks are not needed after vaccinations. Even the CDC guidance was not reassuring enough. Polling on May 20, 2021, showed that only 24 percent of Democrats, 32 percent of independents, and 53 percent of Republicans said they "Strongly Approve" of the CDC's decision to end the mask mandate for those fully vaccinated against COVID-19.

As this book went to press, another mask study appeared. A randomized study of villages in Bangladesh was reported, where some villages were instructed to wear masks and others were not. In that study, the benefit of community masking was reported on limiting symptomatic, antibody-positive COVID illnesses to people, whether or not those tested wore masks, as opposed to the Denmark study proving that masks do not protect mask wearers. This study had two main findings: 1) Cloth masks do not significantly reduce symptomatic antibody-positive COVID disease in any age group; and 2) Surgical masking in villages showed an 11 percent decrease in symptomatic antibody-positive COVID patients, but only in those over fifty. The study had several flaws. If masks were the cause of the decrease, why would that only be in patients over fifty years of age? People in every younger decile showed no significant reduction.

Should that not prompt the idea that older people had a different reason to account for that, since we know that every age group in the village experienced the same impact from others masking? The study tested only for antibodies—did these people become antibody-positive during the study, or were those antibodies pre-existing from a prior infection, even before the study? No testing for virus was performed, so the infection per se was not tested. Only 40 percent of symptomatic agreed to testing for antibodies—that introduced selection bias. Antibody testing has significant false positives and false negatives—would that eliminate all the statistical significance in that one age group, too? And logically, if less than half of villagers in the mask-wearing villages actually wore masks, would that account for significantly fewer symptomatic cases, when we know that masks do not even protect mask wearers themselves? No doubt, the public desperately wants at least one study, some direct evidence, after eighteen months of believing in the efficacy of masks despite all evidence to the contrary. That study is confirmatory that cloth masks are not effective in any aspect of this disease, and it explains again how population masks are not effective at stopping or eliminating COVID-19.

Meanwhile there is reason to anticipate the obsession with masks will continue. During the pandemic, one near uniformity became apparent—influenza essentially disappeared, so claims were made that mask usage eliminated influenza. No one seems to care about the fact that masks do not work for influenza. No one seems to ask why, if masks were so effective in eliminating influenza, they did not stop massive surges in COVID in those same states and nations. No one cares that even in countries without significant mask usage—like Sweden—influenza still disappeared

Ironically, Dr. Fauci had it exactly right back in March 2020 when he said, "There's no reason to be walking around with a mask." He explained some of the science in his own, now-uncovered emails. The subsequent evidence and the best quality scientific research only further confirmed that masks are not effective in preventing the spread of infection from SARS2.

Bottom line: widespread mask usage does not protect mask wearers and does not effectively stop infection from SARS2. And that's the science.

Lockdowns—Reality Matters

Health and Human Services Secretary Alex Azar declared a public health emergency for the United States on January 31, 2020. On March 13, 2020, the White House declared a national state of emergency. America's government leaders embarked on a draconian policy of shutting down society. Restrictions included stay-at-home orders, limits on family visits and group activities, business restrictions and school closures, medical care shutdowns, constraints on personal movement, quarantines, and travel bans—that defines lockdowns. Put forth as a temporary fifteen- or thirty-day closure, the stated goal was to "flatten the curve" of hospitalizations. At the time, the action seemed logical and well-intended. Slow the time line of illness so hospitals could avoid overcrowding and cope with the increasing numbers needing COVID-19 care. That would also allow mobilization of resources, including personnel, beds, and equipment, to those parts of the country where needed most. It would provide extra time to produce tests and protective and medical equipment, and to allow scientists and companies to start developing new drugs and vaccines. Most people accepted the temporary shutdown, given the level of danger implied by the earliest information about the virus.

The policy goal then shifted. No longer was it "flatten the curve." Drs. Fauci and Birx succeeded in convincing America's decision-makers to implement blunt, extremely harsh policies that considered only one specific disease, rather than the whole of health. Those policies were also immoral, because the consequences would fall disproportionately on poor, minority populations and others of low socio-economic status. Instead of concentrating resources on protecting the only group at high risk to die and avoiding serious damage to everyone else, an unfocused and reckless response was broadly instituted. Nearly all US governors implemented and continued those lockdowns throughout 2020 and beyond. Many leaders in other countries did the same.

To be clear, lockdowns were not "due to the virus." To the contrary, lockdowns were voluntarily imposed. They represent decisions that were consciously made. Lockdown harms are not "from the pandemic." Those harms are due to decisions of people in power.

In order to convince the population to acquiesce to such an extreme policy, public health leaders and politicians willingly instilled enormous fear into the public. After months of societal shutdown and hundreds of thousands of deaths before I arrived, I personally sat incredulously as I listened to Dr. Fauci state his opinion in a late August 2020 Task Force meeting. He insisted that Americans were not yet afraid enough. I distinctly asked for clarification of his statement to be sure I heard it correctly. He replied, "Yes, they need to be more afraid." Using emotional distress as a tool to ensure greater adherence to government policy is immoral in public health, yet fear was consciously leveraged by those most influencing the citizenry.

Despite decades of research on the lives lost from severe unemployment and easily obtainable data quantifying health harms from missed medical care, most health economists and social scientists remained quiet. In May 2020, I coauthored a simple column with John Birge of the University of Chicago, Ralph Keeney of Duke University and University of Southern California, and Alex Lipton of Hebrew University of Jerusalem. Considering only losses of life from a small set of missed health care and unemployment, we conservatively estimated the US lockdown was already responsible for at least 700,000 lost years-of-life every month, or about 1.5 million through only May 2020—about double the COVID-19 total in the US at that point of 800,000 lost years of life.

This is the legacy of those who advocated, imposed, and maintained lockdowns:

- Half of the 650,000 cancer patients skipped chemotherapy during the first months of lockdown.

- Forty percent of stroke patients and half of heart attack patients were so afraid they did not call an ambulance; in March-April 2020, New York City alone had a 400 percent increase in deaths from non-COVID heart disease.

- Organ transplants from living donors were down 85 percent from the same period the last year.

- About 46 percent of the top six cancers were not diagnosed during the first four months of the shutdown—these cancers will present for care in later stages, and many people will die.

- Two-thirds to over 80 percent of cancer screenings were skipped in the first three months, including 70 percent of colonoscopies and 67 percent of mammograms. Over nine months, 750,000 to over 1,000,000 new US cancer cases went undetected.

- Severe child abuse cases brought to ERs skyrocketed by 35 percent, brought in by parents who thought they killed their own children.

- Most childhood vaccinations were skipped, generating an impending future health disaster.

- Over the next fifteen years, the unemployment "shock" alone, according to a NBER study, will generate an increased death rate and reduced life expectancy disproportionately affecting African-Americans and women. That computes into a staggering

890,000 extra American deaths—*from the lockdown, not the virus.*

The media and our expert class remained silent as non-COVID deaths from the lockdown were piling up. During the first two months of the pandemic, *more than one-third of our nation's extra deaths were not due to COVID-19.* In fourteen states, more than 50 percent of excess deaths were not attributable to COVID-19 but instead were collateral damage from the lockdowns; these states included California (55 percent of excess deaths) and Texas (64 percent of excess deaths).

On November 2, 2020, I tweeted some eye-opening statistics from CDC data. The death toll continued to mount—and a substantial share was not from the virus. For those sixty-five and older, 39 percent of excess deaths were from causes other than COVID-19. For those aged twenty-five to forty-four, a shocking 77 percent of excess deaths—more than three of four—were not from COVID. These death tolls in the United States were *caused by the lockdowns—not by the virus*—but went virtually unspoken by the Task Force and in the media.

Lockdowns also inflicted tremendous psychological damage, especially harming America's children and younger generation:

- At least one adverse mental health symptom in almost three-fourths of those aged eighteen to twenty-four, college-aged Americans, at the end of June 2020.

- One in four US college-aged kids, ages eighteen to twenty-four, considered suicide after the initial three-month lockdown and as of February 2021 are more than twice as likely as all adults to report new or increased drug use (25 percent vs. 13 percent) or recent suicidal thoughts (26 percent vs. 11 percent).

- Deaths from drug overdoses skyrocketed to 93,331, a record, the sharpest annual increase (30 percent) in at least three decades.

- Hundreds of thousands of child abuse cases in the US were hidden in just the first two months of school closures, since schools are the number one agency where abuse is noticed.

- Doctor visits by teenagers for self-harm—behaviors like slashing wrists, burns, and self-mutilation—tripled in the fall of 2020.

- Suicide attempts among girls ages twelve to seventeen were 50.6 percent higher than they were during the same period in 2019.

- Fifty-two percent of college-aged Americans had a significant, *unwanted* weight gain during the lockdown—and that weight gain averaged a shocking twenty-eight pounds.

- By March 2021, a full 50 percent of those eighteen to twenty-four said they "felt nervous" about *any* future social interaction.

As opposed to the media's false dichotomy to demonize those opposing prolonged lockdowns as "choosing the economy over lives," ending the lockdowns and reopening society is more accurately "saving lives by saving the economy"—especially for the poor and working class. While the elites were "doing their share" on Zoom meetings and telecommuting, the middle and lower classes were subjected to extra exposure to the virus. It is they who worked in the "essential" jobs as defined by the elites—supplying food and other needs in shops, delivering online orders to homes, picking up garbage in neighborhoods, and providing transportation when needed. The lockdowns were not only a luxury of the rich, they were also an abuse of the disadvantaged.

Loss of jobs hit low-wage earners the hardest. In the US, by May 2020, according to data from Harvard and Brown, their unemployment reached over 36 percent—more than triple the 11 percent job loss felt by the top one-quarter of wage earners. As of March 31, 2021, low-wage unemployment remains a massive 24 percent. High-wage earners? Their employment *increased* by 2.4 percent over the pre-pandemic figure.

*   *   *   *   *

It must not be overlooked that American policies impacted more than just Americans. The pronouncements of America's leaders likely also influenced other public health leaders. Additionally, a shutdown of the US is inextricably linked to foreign countries via the interconnected economy. And critical health supplies and services were suspended and resources diverted—all to stop COVID-19:

- Ninety-seven million more people in 2020 were thrown into extreme poverty, according to June 2021 World Bank estimates—that means living on less than $1.90 per day, total.

- Four hundred thousand new deaths from tuberculosis will occur in the next year alone, and over 1 million in the next three years.

- Tens of thousands additional malaria deaths in babies occurred in 2020, due to interruption of resources.

- A hundred million or more children were exposed to sexual abuse and exploitation, violence, genital mutilation, and childhood pregnancies due to school closures.

- More than 1.5 billion children were shut out of their education, and 369 million children worldwide did not receive basic nutritional needs because school meals were unavailable.

- In Bangladesh, the backbone of their economy, garment manufacturing, was virtually shut down by cancellation of 900 million pieces of garments worth $2.9 billion in spring 2020 alone. That industry supplies 4.1 million families with their only income.

- Thirty million of India's citizens were thrown back from middle class to poverty this year alone.

- When GDP falls in poor countries, life expectancy falls dramatically. The African Development Bank showed a collapse in African GDPs, with several countries seeing GDP losses of more than 8 percent, likely underestimates of the impact.

Did the Lockdowns Stop COVID-19 Cases and Deaths?

The disastrous consequences of the lockdowns cannot be denied by any honest appraisal. The burden of proof is on the lockdown policy to have saved more lives. That leaves the question—Did the lockdowns stop COVID-19? Did lockdowns reduce the deaths during the pandemic?

All scientists recognize that it may be difficult to compare COVID-19 data internationally. A 2021 RAND institute study by Mahshid Abir found major differences in reporting COVID information from tests, hospitalizations, and even deaths.

Some countries required a positive SARS2 virus test to call a death as being from COVID. Others relied only on symptoms, even without a COVID-positive test. Some countries had far more widespread testing programs than others, or tested only sick individuals, important because half or more of infected people are without symptoms. If tests were heavily relied on, then the technique of the test also mattered. For instance, the UK used PCR tests with "cycle thresholds" of forty-five, a number so high that inactive virus from weeks earlier was detected—many patients may not have had active illness for weeks, if ever. Some countries counted a death as being from COVID based solely on a positive test, even if that patient had no symptoms of COVID. One Stanford study confirmed the misclassification among 117 pediatric cases, all categorized as "hospitalized for COVID." About 45 percent could not have been due to COVID—*they had zero symptoms of the illness*, even though they had a positive test for the virus. Similar findings were reported in a separate large study, where 40 percent of patients were incidentally positive on PCR tests but were not truly ill with COVID.

A second major difficulty in comparisons is that populations differ in their risk to COVID. Each country has stark differences in age demographics, obesity, or diabetes. Certain countries are more isolated geographically and have different climates, lifestyle factors, and proportions of rural or urban living. While it is not known with certainty, preexisting immunity from past exposure to other coronaviruses may have limited some countries' harms from SARS2.

From the growing body of scientific research, there is little evidence that lockdowns were successful in saving lives or preventing cases of COVID-19:

- Quentin De Larochelambert in November 2020 concluded, "Stringency of the measures settled to fight pandemia, including lockdown, did not appear to be linked with death rate" on a multi-country evaluation of the 2020 lockdowns.

- Christian Bjørnskov in March 2021 concluded, "Comparing weekly mortality in 24 European countries, the findings in this paper suggest that more severe lockdown policies have not been associated with lower mortality. In other words, the lockdowns have not worked as intended."

- Bendavid, Oh, Bhattacharya, and Ioannidis in January 2021 compared lockdowns (mandatory stay-at-home orders and business closures) to less restrictive policies in ten countries (England, France, Germany, Iran, Italy, Netherlands, Spain, South Korea, Sweden, and the United States) on the growth of cases in the initial wave of 2020. They concluded, "(We) do not find significant benefits on case growth of more restrictive NPIs (non-pharmaceutical interventions, i.e., lockdowns)." According to Ioannidis, the lockdowns were "usually harmful," "pro-contagion."

- Agrawal in June 2021 found that lockdown policies in forty-three countries and in US states led to *more excess deaths*:

  o With longer shelter-in-place orders, *more* excess deaths occurred

  o With faster lockdowns, *more* excess deaths occurred.

  o In the forty-three countries with available data, excess deaths were falling before lockdowns, but *once lockdowns were instituted, the death toll began rising.*

    o In the US states, deaths *increased once lockdowns were implemented.*

In that analysis, the only countries where lockdowns reduced excess mortality were islands—Australia, New Zealand, and Malta—and the only state was the island state of Hawaii.

As for the cases within the US, America has one very enlightening internal comparison: that between Florida and California. This comparison is made as of the end of spring, 2021.

Florida is unique among all large, diverse states in the US in that it did not follow the Fauci-Birx prolonged lockdown pathway. Governor DeSantis chose to use a focused protection strategy, resisting calls for issuing mask mandates and prolonged lockdowns.

DeSantis aggressively protected Florida's nursing home residents. First, on March 15, he banned all visitations to long-term care facilities. Second, he issued an order forbidding COVID-positive patients from reentering nursing homes after hospital discharge. Third, he established COVID-dedicated senior facilities all over the state. That directly contrasted with governors in New York (March 25, 2020), Pennsylvania (March 18, 2020), Michigan (April 15, 2020), New Jersey (March 31, 2020), and California (April 10 and May 15, 2020), whose policies potentially introduced the infection into the deadliest possible environment.

After initial closures, DeSantis reopened all Florida schools for in-person learning by August 2020. On September 1, he said, "We will never do any of these lockdowns again," and ended business closures, discarded mobility restrictions, and eliminated mask mandates. In October, he lifted visitation restrictions to long-term care facilities, with guidelines. Almost all other US governors instead maintained school and business closures, mask mandates, restrictions on personal activities, and other shutdowns.

Florida did not eliminate cases, hospitalizations, or deaths, and more will follow, given that the virus will not disappear. Predictably, a seasonal surge in Florida and the southern states is underway at the time of this writing. Over 37,000 Floridians deaths have been attributed to COVID-19. Florida, even with its large, high-risk population of elderly in 4,000 long-term care facilities, outperformed most states that maintained societal closures.

- Florida outperformed the overall USA for COVID deaths per capita.

- Florida outperformed twenty-five individual states (lockdown states) in COVID deaths per capita.

- Florida outperformed forty states in overall age-adjusted COVID mortality.

- Florida outperformed forty states in age-adjusted COVID mortality for those sixty-five-plus years old, the high-risk group.

- Florida outperformed—by 40 percent—the overall United States age-adjusted COVID mortality.

- Florida outperformed two-thirds of states in excess mortality increase (percent increase in all deaths over a non-pandemic year).

- Florida outperformed—by 24 percent—the overall United States excess mortality increase.

How did Florida compare to other large states with similar urban-rural populations and diversity?

- Florida ranks number one of the ten largest states in lowest excess mortality.

- Florida ranks number one of the ten largest states in lowest age-adjusted mortality for those aged sixty-five-plus.

- Florida ranks number one of the ten largest states in lowest age-adjusted mortality for all ages.

For further illumination Florida should be compared to another large, diverse, mixed urban-rural state with a similar climate—California. Florida has the fifth oldest population in the country, while California is much younger, with the nation's seventh youngest population. California implemented and maintained very stringent lockdowns.

- *Florida did better than California in protecting its citizens from dying.* The overall age-adjusted per-capita COVID mortality rate in Florida is 118 per 100,000, while it is 168 per 100,000 people in California. California's excess mortality rate was 58 percent higher than Florida's (27 percent versus 17 percent).

- *Florida did better at protecting its minorities.* Bhattacharya calculated that through March 28, 2021, Hispanics in LA suffered the worst of the pandemic, with a death rate of 338 per 100,000. Black and White residents had 188 and 119 deaths per 100,000, respectively. In Florida, by contrast, Black and Hispanic populations died at lower rates than the White population.

- *Florida did better at protecting jobs for lower-income people.* According to Harvard and Brown University research, of March 31, 2021, employment for low-wage earners in California was down 38.3 percent. In Florida, employment for low-wage earners was increased by 0.4 percent.

Once vaccinations became available, Governor DeSantis continued adhering to the focused protection model. He rejected CDC guidance and instead put elderly at the very top of vaccination prioritization. Even if Floridians behaved in some ways similarly to people under mandates, they and their children did not suffer from the severe harms of school and work closures. And fewer died.

Bottom line: Lockdowns did not stop the virus or save lives. Massive lives were lost because of the lockdowns. Focused protection was the safer and more ethical strategy. "Long lockdown" is far worse than "long COVID." It's not even close. And that's the science

* * * * *

Throughout the pandemic, owing to the power of the media and the active suppression of science itself, the public was manipulated to think that everyone in science naturally agreed with the mandates and harsh restrictions of lockdowns. But scientific truth is not declared by consensus. It arises from research, critical thinking, and debate, not groupthink and censure of alternative views. All legitimate policy scholars should, today, be openly reexamining lockdowns, the policies that severely harmed America's families and children, while failing to protect the elderly. That damage will go on for years, perhaps decades.

There was a safer, more logical, more scientific alternative—targeted protection of the vulnerable. That strategy saved lives and avoided the catastrophic harms of prolonged lockdowns. Public health policies should always consider the impact on whole health, not just stopping the spread of a single disease, and the harms and benefits of those policies. By airing the facts in this book that have been ignored, denied, censored, or distorted, it is my hope that we will never let this tragic, misguided policy happen again.

CODA
1984 Meets Cancel Culture

I arrived in Washington in the middle of a crisis, in a heavily polarized nation burdened by fear, encountering a hostile media inflamed during an election year. I learned quickly, abruptly, what was meant by a "Washington Welcome." Once I was unveiled as an advisor to President Trump, my eyes were opened by the realization that even in this once-in-a-lifetime crisis, the dissemination of truth is not the priority of American media.

That is not an overstatement, and it is dangerous to dismiss it as hyperbole. Or maybe that doesn't surprise anyone but me. A truth-seeking, honest press was always one of the most crucial differences between the United States and countries we proudly stood in distinction from—the USSR, Russia, China, North Korea, Cuba. Thinking through the reality of what we were all told during this pandemic, and how it was crafted by the media, should send chills through every American. I am still reeling from knowing it, even though I now expect it.

Tactics were somewhat different between legacy and social media platforms, given that Big Tech can literally delete and censor with impunity. That said, news shows and digital print can also distort and lie with impunity. But it was not just the content of the media; it was the way it was delivered that influenced the public. Nowadays, misleading stories are easier to invent and quicker to amplify on both platforms.

Despite what many might assume, American media proved to be a uniquely unreliable purveyor of information. American media stood out in editorializing the pandemic, worse than all other English-language news sources. The top-level evidence was their extremist slant on all news related to the pandemic. By end of summer 2020, no end was in sight to the pandemic or the lockdowns. Almost two hundred Americans had died, and the public was understandably fearful. More than nine million articles had been published from January 31 through July 31, 2020. On every important issue, America's media was pushing a biased narrative:

- America's reporting was alone in virtually always being negative—nine of ten stories by all of America's major media outlets were negative in tone. Fox News articles were as negative as those from CNN. The comparison? Outside the US, the major news stories were negative only half the time.

- On the vaccine—the most important hope of almost everyone—America's major media were particularly negative. Vaccine stories in the US major media were 45 percentage points more likely to be negative than vaccine stories in the non-US media.

- American media intentionally omitted or delayed reporting positive news.

   o Even when new COVID cases were *declining* in the US, articles describing *increasing* cases outnumbered stories of decreasing cases by a factor of more than five to one.

- Work on a vaccine was reported on February 18, 2020, by the UK's news, but Fox News, CNN, the *New York Times*, and the *Washington Post* did not begin any coverage of Professor Gilbert's COVID-19 vaccine until late April.

- The earliest available report about a vaccine development in the US major media, dated April 23, began with England's chief medical officer, Chris Whitty, saying that the probability of having a vaccine "anytime in the next calendar year" is "incredibly small." (Note: the vaccine was announced just over six months later, and Americans began receiving injected vaccine in December 2020.)

- America's media created a frightening, false narrative about schools with biased news. While the world's data was overwhelmingly positive about schools reopening, 90 percent of school reopening articles from US mainstream media were negative; only half (56 percent) were negative in other countries. (Note: Europe's schools were widely opened for fall 2020, whereas only 18 percent of US schools were in-person and 60 percent were virtual-only.)

It is undeniable that this was intentional—obviously, the media decides what and how to report. Might the negative presentation have been politically motivated, to heighten fear and a feeling of scandalous incompetence about the Trump administration just a few months ahead of the election? Regardless of the true motive, it did not serve the public well. That flow of overwhelmingly negative stories, introduced tremendous anxiety and damaged the mental health of the public. No doubt it impacted policy, too. By January 2021, the CDC advised Americans, "Take breaks from watching, reading, or listening to news stories." That was good advice, but few took it.

A central claim of his media opponents to discredit President Trump, voiced almost on a daily basis, was "He doesn't listen to the science!" If true, then that would be totally unacceptable, a disqualifier for anyone in a leadership position at the height of a deadly health crisis. That claim, whether or not truly believed by the accusers, led in turn to a key tactic. If anyone with legitimate scientific, medical, or academic credentials put forth evidence that happened to bolster the points of the president, they too must be destroyed.

After months of highlighting the president's misstatements and playing up conflicts with Dr. Fauci and a host of talking heads, the media encountered a new obstacle to their mission. I was suddenly standing next to the president in the press briefing room in August. I had seen the hate in the president's press briefings on television, but I was struck right away by the undignified, unprofessional behavior of the press corps in the room. Often off-camera, they hurled heinous accusations ("WHEN ARE YOU GOING TO STOP LYING?" and "YOU KILLED HUNDREDS OF THOUSANDS OF PEOPLE!!") at the president in the briefing room with undisguised venom. That behavior didn't even include how little most reporters actually understood about the questions they asked, despite their displays of aggressiveness and bravado in posing them.

My appearance created a problem for the media. If a highly qualified health policy scholar and medical scientist from Stanford was advising President Trump, that would muddy their claim. The fact that I espoused policies, backed by evidence, that aligned with what the president had stated made it even worse. Instead of conflicting with the president's desire to reopen or undermining him like the media's favorite Task Force members who pushed for continued lockdowns, I had the audacity to cite a stream of scientific evidence that supported reopening schools and businesses. I put forth legitimate data that questioned their orthodoxies about immune protection, risks to children, masks, and the failure of lockdowns. Under no circumstances could that be permitted to stand.

Almost immediately after being introduced by the president at his August 10 press briefing, a coordinated effort began within the mainstream media to discredit me. By distorting my words and using straw-man arguments and personal attacks, the tabloid press—the *Washington Post*, CNN, and others formerly regarded as legitimate news outlets—intentionally and maliciously tried to harm my reputation and delegitimize me. Kushner had warned me about this back in July, and he had his own experience with it. Admittedly, though, the intensity of it caught me by surprise. I had agreed to help, even though I knew half the country considered this president radioactive. "OK," I thought, "I am a pretty confident person." In my decades in academics, I had never once been worried, let alone questioned, about my claim to expertise. As I told the *Wall Street Journal* in their September profile of me soon after the press mauling had begun, "I am pretty comfortable with my CV." Not to mention that I knew what I was talking about. I had been working with the top epidemiologists at Stanford and had analyzed the data in excruciating detail for months. Hey, after all, I had even convinced my skeptical wife by then!

The press adopted a two-pronged approach. Legacy media deployed distortions and falsifications with impunity, while political talk show hacks went on irresponsible, low-level rants filled with lies that occasionally caught my eye while facing large-screen TVs during breakfast at the hotel. I wasn't much for breakfast, anyway.

It was not just the conventional, or "legacy," media that aggressively tried to demonize me and my views. Social media, particularly Twitter, YouTube, and Facebook, was actively suffocating voices, including mine, that dissented from the accepted COVID narrative. By August, Facebook told the *Washington Post* they had taken down seven million posts "for spreading coronavirus misinformation." Meanwhile, Wikipedia crafted smears and distortions of my background and then locked it to edits.

Three examples stand out:

- On September 11, YouTube suddenly pulled down a lengthy interview I had done on June 23 back at Stanford, months before named as advisor to the president. In that episode of Peter Robinson's *Uncommon Knowledge*, I focused on the safety of school reopening and the extremely low risk for children from COVID-19, including the low risk of transmission from children to adults—all known at the time of the interview and backed by an over-whelming body of scientific data. That interview was suddenly removed with notification that the video "violates our guidelines." Hoover was later permitted to repost the video, but YouTube added the following comment: "YouTube does not allow content that spreads medical misinformation that contradicts the World Health Organization (WHO) or local health authorities' medical information about COVID-19, including on methods to prevent, treat, or diagnose COVID-19 and means of transmission of COVID-19."

- On October 18, Twitter blocked my account. I had posted a multipart tweet the day before question-ing the efficacy of masks, listing cities and states where cases surged through masking, and quoting authoritative data, including CDC, WHO, and Ox-ford. I also reiterated warnings to observe estab-lished mitigation protocols including masking and social distancing when appropriate. Yet the mes-sage provoked prompt censorship and a temporary ban from Twitter.

The news erupted, as did the fervor of those who were forced to hear what they considered anathema. Friends told me that to question the efficacy of general population masks in this pandemic would be the equivalent of the heresy of Galileo. There was no way to deny it—right here in the USA, the freedom to express a valid scientific viewpoint had been obliterated. In what free society would it be disallowed to state scientific evidence?

I quickly clicked the link to accept their censorship, a necessary part of my reinstatement. The next morning, I posted a simple tweet without any mention of masks:

> "The Party told you to reject the evidence of your eyes and ears.
>
> It was their final, most essential command."
>
> "And if all others accepted the lie which the Party imposed—if all records told the same tale—
>
> then the lie passed into history and became truth."
>
> *George Orwell, 1984*

The tweet went viral, eventually totaling about four million views. Twitter comments erupted with a mix of support and condemnation. Demands for condemnation of me came on cable TV and news outlets. CNN and their cadre of science-deniers, many of whom were quite comfortable posing as experts, demanded that I must be condemned for this heresy. The pushback was intense and widespread, including from professors at elite institutions.

It did not matter that the mask quotes were right off of the very health agencies they relied on for their own views—this was cognitive dissonance in action. Charts filled with evidence of cases bursting through masks in dozens of cities, states, and countries were simply not acknowledged. Perhaps rooted in repudiation of President Trump's less-than-full endorsement of masks, people were now full-blown zealots about masks, evidence be damned! They were so deeply, so emotionally, committed to the power of masks that facts literally did not matter to these people. Groupthink had firmly taken hold—and views to the contrary must not even be visible, according to the powerful arbiters of America's speech.

- On March 18, 2021, Florida Governor DeSantis assembled an expert panel to discuss the pandemic, including natural immunity, masks, lockdowns, and school closures. Four of us participated—myself, Kulldorff, Bhattacharya, and Gupta. In the discussion, Bhattacharya stated, "The evidence is clear. The lockdowns have not stopped the spread of the disease in any measurable way." About masks, Kulldorff responded that "children should not wear face masks, no. They don't need it for their own protection and they don't need it for protecting other people, either." Asked if there is any basis for masks outdoors, Bhattacharya said, "The answer is no." The panel video was taken down, censored by YouTube through its "medical misinformation policy." On April 8, 2021, the Wall Street Journal wrote in "YouTube's Assault on COVID Accountability" that "it's chilling that Google's YouTube appears to be systematically undermining the ability to access material in the public interest." Governor DeSantis soon followed up with another panel, specifically to highlight the inappropriate, indeed dangerous, attempt by big tech to selectively stop the public from hearing information from experts that the censors oppose.

The danger of censoring the president's advisor about the pandemic, *during the pandemic*, was not lost on some thinking journalists, who pointed out the dangers:

- *The Federalist's* Jonathan Tobin wrote, "YouTube's arbitrary censorship of Dr. Atlas ought to be the straw that breaks the camel's back concerning its ability to shut down speech about COVID-19 issues." He continued, "Atlas didn't deny the seriousness of the disease or the need to act to prevent its spread—he merely questioned the efficacy of broad lockdowns."

- The *Wall Street Journal* editorial board observed, "The Atlas interview was posted in June, yet YouTube only removed it in September. The public can be forgiven for wondering if Dr. Atlas's appointment as a White House coronavirus adviser last month has made him a political target. A group of Stanford faculty published an open letter sliming their former colleague last week, and the video came down two days later."

I interviewed on Tucker Carlson's Fox show that same week and said something that should never need to be stated out loud. "We ought to be able to accept differences in science (interpretations) and go forward and prove it." That's the essence of science, isn't it?

What came as an even more powerful shock was that medical science and academia were now as broken as the media, undeniably infected with politics and a desire to censor opposing views. The parallels are striking, extending to the tactics of brazen intimidation and cancellation of anyone countering the orthodoxy. Faculty at many universities overtly intimidated those with views contrary to their own, leaving many afraid to speak up. That intimidation has been quite effective—I know, having received hundreds of emails from scientists and policy scholars from all over the country, indeed all over the world, telling me they are afraid to come forward. Even a number of infectious disease experts at Stanford were afraid and remain reluctant to step forward publicly.

The free exchange of ideas—the scientific process itself that generates the desperately needed solutions for our nation's crises—has not been allowed by the science community itself in this pandemic. False declarations of "consensus" and vicious demonization of those with alternative views suddenly replaced critical analysis and debate over data. The outright ignoring of contradictory but superior research, the distortion of others' interpretations, and the refusal to admit error became standard.

One vehicle for the suffocation of science was our most important source of research knowledge—the science journals and academia. Politically motivated professors at elite universities and some of the world's most influential medical science journals abrogated their responsibility to the world and instead became opinionated vehicles for censorship and intimidation. Top medical journals suppressed data by omission in an effort to conjure up their chosen "consensus." Major journals shockingly published opinion pieces in an attempt to intimidate and "cancel" the research and scientific interpretations of the evidence pointed out by me, the acclaimed scientists authoring the Great Barrington Declaration, and other top experts.

- In July 2020, the *New England Journal of Medicine* published an article on 'reopening primary schools during the pandemic.' Amazingly, it did not even mention the evidence from the only major Western country that kept schools open throughout the pandemic, Sweden. As Harvard's Martin Kulldorff put it, "That is like evaluating a new drug while ignoring data from the placebo control group."

- In February 2020, the influential journal Lancet published a remarkable letter signed by prominent virologists and other scientists. The authors began by lauding China for their "rapid, open, and transparent sharing of data"—even though the world knew that China delayed warning the world about the early COVID cases, forbade an open exploration of the Wuhan lab, and subsequently destroyed critical evidence that could have helped identify the origin of the virus. The authors undermined the public's trust in science itself by abusing their platform as a tool of intimidation.

- The scientists wrote, "We stand together to strongly condemn conspiracy theories [italics added] suggesting that COVID-19 does not have a natural origin. Scientists from multiple countries have published and analysed genomes of the causative agent, severe acute respiratory syndrome coronavirus 2 (SARS-CoV-2), and they overwhelmingly conclude that this coronavirus originated in wildlife." They then explicitly, and shockingly, called for "unity"—an unheard of plea from scientists interested in research-driven conclusions. It was an unbridled attempt to marginalize and preempt any scientist who might show contrary evidence about the origin of the virus—evidence that we now know was present even then, as shown by the trove of Fauci emails later exposed under FOIA.

- In October 2020, *Lancet* published an extraordinarily misleading opinion piece in which group of scientists and professors tried to force their opinions, some of which were contrary to scientific evidence about immunity, onto the public as some sort of settled consensus. As Kulldorff and Bhattacharya pointed out, the *Lancet* authors falsely stated that "there is no evidence for lasting protective immunity to SARS-CoV-2 following natural infection."

The *Lancet* piece tried to demonize the authors of the Great Barrington Declaration, wrongly claiming that they advocated letting the infection "spread freely until population immunity was achieved"—which would cause massive deaths.

- In February 2021, *JAMA* published a defamatory attack on me by three unhinged Stanford professors. Citing lay newspapers as their references, they falsely claimed that "nearly all public health experts were concerned that [Atlas's] recommendations could lead to tens of thousands (or more) of unnecessary deaths in the US alone." As pointed out by Joel Zinberg, the Great Barrington Declaration is "far closer to the one condemned in the *JAMA* article than anything [Atlas] said." Yet that policy declaration was coauthored by some of the world's leading medical scientists and epidemiologists from Stanford, Harvard, and Oxford and had already been signed by over fifty thousand medical and public-health practitioners. The editor of *JAMA* refused to publish rebuttals written by highly respected medical scientists backing up my scientific analyses—I know, because I was contacted by the authors after their rejection.

Scientists and the media shared the same strategy: seek out and destroy all who dared dissent from the accepted narrative, and delegitimize everything uttered by President Trump and all who agreed with him. Instead of rethinking failed policies and admitting their errors, these scientists chose to employ smears and organized rebukes against those of us who disagreed with what was implemented and who dared to help the president they despised. One thing was clear—everything President Trump said about the pandemic must be discredited, delegitimized, vilified, and maligned.

- When President Trump posited that the virus might have leaked out of the Wuhan virology research lab, that obvious possibility was strongly denied by America's lead pandemic advisor, when it could not have possibly been known, and was derided as a conspiracy theory by respected scientists in one of the world's most prestigious scientific journals.

- When President Trump prematurely claimed that hydroxychloroquine was an effective treatment, that drug—a drug used by hundreds of millions with a sixty-five-year track record of proven safety—was absurdly claimed to be dangerous. As a result, urgently needed clinical trials by the NIH and FDA were never performed. In another unprecedented move, doctors were blocked from prescribing the drug, even though prescribing any other approved drug for an off-label use was routine.

- When President Trump called for ending school closures, scientists and doctors deliberately denied a trove of compelling data, falsely claiming that children were dangerous vectors of the disease and were themselves at significant risk, as were their teachers.

- When President Trump called for diligently protecting the vulnerable while ending lockdowns and reopening businesses, public health and science leaders misrepresented the proposal, ignored the evidence, and denied the scientific studies to frighten the public.

- When President Trump announced that under Operation Warp Speed, life-saving vaccines were going to be available before the end of 2020, scientists and public health officials repeatedly denounced that possibility as a lie, undermined public confidence in the safety of any vaccine developed by the Trump administration, and the announcement of the vaccine's effectiveness was delayed until after the election.

To this day, most people do not fully understand the policy advice from those of us who advocated a safer, more targeted strategy and who made the case that prolonged lockdowns were the incorrect policy. Much of that confusion is owed to the tragic success of those who control the information. The public has been manipulated by a powerful coalition of elites in politics, academia, media, and big tech. Two central untruths were thrust upon a naive public to discredit the call to end the draconian lockdown policies. Neither of those arguments had any scientific foundation.

The first lie arose near the beginning of lockdowns. Lockdown advocates cast those calling for reopening as "choosing the economy over lives." That false dichotomy was set up in order to shame and intimidate scientists opposing the lockdowns. In most cases, the strategy worked.

The second tactic was to squash the opposition to lockdowns by instilling fear and demonizing those calling for focused protection with reopening. That was effectively done with straw-man arguments—by misrepresenting the focused protection policy and then arguing against that false definition. Lockdown advocates misrepresented targeted protection as letting the infection spread freely in a so-called "let it rip" or "herd immunity" strategy. This tactic was deployed against both me and the signers of the Great Barrington Declaration.

As time went on, the false notion that any mention of herd immunity endorsed a reckless and dangerous strategy of encouraging infection to spread took on a life of its own. It became the most weaponized term in the pandemic, a tool to quite effectively demonize all those who decried the failures and harms of the lockdowns while proposing a safer, more effective, targeted protection. Today, as the world still struggles with the biological truth of the importance of natural immunity as part of herd immunity, I contemplate why it was viewed as some sort of diabolical term. But it's clear to see why it was employed by those clinging to lockdowns at all costs. Casting herd immunity as reckless and dangerous was unethical, but ultimately even more effective than simple character assassination for a political purpose. Of all the cynical ways to manipulate people, fear was their best way to maintain lockdowns, despite the massive destruction from lockdowns that regular people saw before their own eyes.

The herd immunity frenzy was only part of a broader plan. In the eyes of elites in science, academia, big tech, media, and politics, further evidence by researchers to support ending lockdowns was the true "danger." Focused protection and reopening would mesh with the opinion of President Trump, and that could not be permitted.

To be sure, misrepresentations about the efficacy of lockdowns were not monopolized by popular media or the public health personalities. Nor were they confined to Twitter, where a number of academics were perversely enjoying their newfound fame with a receptive, impressionable audience. Poorly documented claims about the success of the lockdowns became acceptable to some of the most prestigious scientific journals, as long as it supported their continuation. Perhaps most illustrative was a report in *Nature* in August 2020, which claimed that non-pharmaceutical interventions imposed by eleven European countries saved millions of lives. Two researchers analyzed those claims in *Frontiers in Medicine* in November 2020 and showed that the authors relied on purely circular logic. They also showed the United Kingdom's lockdown was ineffective. Yet the original paper still stands, unretracted, despite its circular reasoning and wholly incorrect conclusions.

Another of many false impressions pushed by lockdown advocates was Sweden's record in the pandemic. Held up as another "let it rip" example, Sweden did not lock down like most other countries in Europe. Instead, Sweden mainly relied on voluntary measures like social distancing, hygiene, and targeted rules that kept schools, restaurants, and businesses largely open. More ironically, Sweden has been held as an exemplar of bad pandemic practice; yet that flies in the face of the evidence. Sweden did poorly in protecting the elderly—more than half the deaths in Stockholm were in nursing homes, for instance. But the story in Sweden is very different from the propaganda pushed in the American media. Overall, the dire projections of death tolls in Sweden never came close to materializing, totaling lower than forecasts by several multiples. Sweden's excess mortality during the pandemic is better than two-thirds of European countries. In a ranking of excess mortality of thirty-one countries in Europe, Sweden ranked ninth best, beating most Western European countries that had all imposed far stricter lockdowns. If harsh isolation and closure strategies of schools, businesses, and healthy people did not save massive numbers of lives, then how will history record the justification for the lockdowns' tolls of destruction on healthy people? As I write this, Sweden has been conspicuously absent in the media. Why? While many European countries are adding restrictions and locking down as cases increase, Sweden is wide open, with businesses, schools, and tourism thriving—with zero COVID deaths per day. Not much exciting to report there. In his understated way, Sweden's chief epidemiologist, Anders Tegnell, recently told Reuters he believed the data raised doubts about the use of lockdowns. "I think people will probably think very carefully about these total shutdowns, how good they really were," he said.

* * * * *

The most off-base attempt to undermine my credibility was not the transparent disregard for my seventeen-year career in health policy and twenty-five-plus years in medical science, while dismissing me as "a radiologist"—a career that I left nearly a decade ago. Nor was it the irrelevant but amusing "accusation" that I am not an epidemiologist. That and other misinformation had some legs, because Trump haters wanted to believe it and because the media, too, engages in herd thinking. But the most harmful distortion to the American public was the *Washington Post* story that claimed that I was advising the president to intentionally let the infection spread as a way to achieve "herd immunity." I never advised that. To the contrary, I called for extra sanitization, social distancing, masks, group limits, testing, and other increased protections to limit the spread and damage from the virus, and to specifically augment protection of those at high risk in dozens of on-the-record presentations, interviews, and written pieces. That reprehensible falsehood generated serious fear in the public. And like the other political attacks in the pandemic, that tool was leveraged by both the media and the scientific community to achieve their goals.

Finally, on October 4, 2020, Martin Kulldorff, Sunetra Gupta, and Jay Bhattacharya—three of the most preeminent epidemiologists and medical scientists in the world—published the Great Barrington Declaration. In it, they called for increasing the focused protection of high-risk individuals and ending the broad lockdowns. That single document will go down as one of the most important publications in the pandemic, as it lent undeniable credibility to focused protection and provided courage to thousands of additional medical scientists and public health leaders to come forward. Here is the text of that document:

The Great Barrington Declaration

As infectious disease epidemiologists and public health scientists we have grave concerns about the damaging physical and mental health impacts of the prevailing COVID-19 policies, and recommend an approach we call Focused Protection.

Coming from both the left and right, and around the world, we have devoted our careers to protecting people. Current lockdown policies are producing devastating effects on short and long-term public health. The results (to name a few) include lower childhood vaccination rates, worsening cardiovascular disease outcomes, fewer cancer screenings and deteriorating mental health – leading to greater excess mortality in years to come, with the working class and younger members of society carrying the heaviest burden. Keeping students out of school is a grave injustice.

Keeping these measures in place until a vaccine is available will cause irreparable damage, with the underprivileged disproportionately harmed.

Fortunately, our understanding of the virus is growing. We know that vulnerability to death from COVID-19 is more than a thousand-fold higher in the old and infirm than the young. Indeed, for children, COVID-19 is less dangerous than many other harms, including influenza.

As immunity builds in the population, the risk of infection to all – including the vulnerable – falls. We know that all populations will eventually reach herd immunity – i.e. the point at which the rate of new infections is stable – and that this can be assisted by (but is not dependent upon) a vaccine. Our goal should therefore be to minimize mortality and social harm until we reach herd immunity.

The most compassionate approach that balances the risks and benefits of reaching herd immunity, is to allow those who are at minimal risk of death to live their lives normally to build up immunity to the virus through natural infection, while better protecting those who are at highest risk. We call this Focused Protection.

Adopting measures to protect the vulnerable should be the central aim of public health responses to COVID-19. By way of example, nursing homes should use staff with acquired immunity and perform frequent testing of other staff and all visitors. Staff rotation should be minimized. Retired people living at home should have groceries and other essentials delivered to their home. When possible, they should meet family members outside rather than inside. A comprehensive and detailed list of measures, including approaches to multi-generational households, can be implemented, and is well within the scope and capability of public health professionals.

Those who are not vulnerable should immediately be allowed to resume life as normal. Simple hygiene measures, such as hand washing and staying home when sick should be practiced by everyone to reduce the herd immunity threshold. Schools and universities should be open for in-person teaching. Extracurricular activities, such as sports, should be resumed. Young low-risk adults should work normally, rather than from home. Restaurants and other businesses should open. Arts, music, sport and other cultural activities should resume. People who are more at risk may participate if they wish, while society as a whole enjoys the protection conferred upon the vulnerable by those who have built up herd immunity.

A barrage of misinformation and ad hominem attacks came forward. None were scientifically sound. And the real goal of the misinformation campaign to discredit all opposing views became visible to the entire world, and was shown to reach all the way to the top.

Less than a week before the election, on October 28, I saw an interview with the future president of the United States, Joe Biden, on CBS's *60 Minutes*. When directly asked about my ideas on the pandemic using focused protection and ending the lockdowns, President Biden said, "Nobody thinks (Atlas) makes any sense. No serious doc in the world." Today, as of June 27, 2021, despite extraordinary attempts by the most powerful elites of society to delegitimize all calls to end the lockdowns and to nullify all data proving its shameful harms, the Great Barrington Declaration calling for focused protection and an end to the lockdowns has been co-signed by 14,794 public health and medical scientists, and 43,575 medical practitioners at the time of this writing. *With all due respect, Mr. President, that's a lot of nobodies.*

However, there was something far more important than any of the negative hit pieces. Something that lies and distortions from hateful people could never overcome. The media, the politicized scientists and health agencies, the university attackers had no idea what was driving me on, in the face of their attempts to discredit and cancel me.

First and foremost, I knew I was right. People were dying from the virus, and the lockdown policies were not preventing the deaths. The simple logic of assuming you could stop the spread of, and some said eliminate, a highly contagious virus by shutting down society after millions had been infected was worse than nonsensical. The idea of stopping all businesses and closing schools while quarantining healthy young people at little risk from a disease in order to protect those aged seventy and over—that is simply irrational. Meanwhile the catastrophic tragedy of the prolonged lockdowns was simply denied by those imposing them. The failure to stop cases and deaths was being ignored. This was active destruction of humanity by decree, and on a massive scale. It was absolutely inconceivable, and it would have been morally wrong, to sit silently and watch such gross incompetence destroy millions of people.

But there was also a more personal inspiration that helped me persevere. My colleagues, top scientists from Stanford, Harvard, and all over the world kept cheering me on with their reassurances that "truth will prevail." The epidemiologists whom I respected the most kept encouraging me. We knew, without a doubt, that we were correct. The data proved it. Fundamentals of biology and infectious disease proved it. Analysis of the harms of missed medical care, psychological damage from school closures and unemployment, and the lives lost from the economic shutdown proved it.

Then there were the contacts from perfect strangers. Throughout my time in Washington, I received a continual stream of emails—hundreds per day, thousands every week. They were overwhelmingly positive, encouraging me to continue. Many were frankly emotional; some were very difficult to read. The came from all over the country. Hundreds were from outside the US—Europe, Canada, Brazil, Asia. Some were from researchers, medical scientists, epidemiologists, computer scientists, and students offering their data and asking for my thoughts or help in getting their studies published. But most were from regular citizens, young and old, mothers and fathers. Many were seniors who knew they were in the high-risk group but were passionately opposed to the lockdowns; they repeatedly told me they did not want to continue living under lockdown conditions, without seeing their grandchildren and loved ones. Reverends, school teachers, school board members, parents, teenagers, and business owners related their personal stories. Some asked questions about data. Some contained very personal details that I could never have anticipated from perfect strangers. Many used words that truly moved me, almost begging me to continue speaking out, pleading with me for their kids, their elderly parents, their students. Some assured me they were praying for me, reminding me that millions more were supporting my efforts to open schools, to end the lockdowns. I still receive many kind and supportive emails today, some from journalists who never even interviewed me. I truly thank them all for their support.

Many painful emails will also forever stand out. They are heartbreaking to reread, but they, too, served as a profound inspiration to me. From what seems like an eternity ago but is just one year, a pediatric ER doctor wrote to tell me that she agreed about reopening schools. She said her Michigan hospital was seeing an explosion of severely beaten kids, some near death. She wrote, "PEM [pediatric emergency medicine] doctors everywhere knew kids would pay the price of unemployed parents staying home too long in the form of hunger and beatings." Several other emails told me to keep speaking out, because their husband or child or elderly parent had just committed suicide from the isolation of the lockdown.

They still remind me of what's really important, and why it's so necessary to stand up and speak for the truth. No matter what.